NEVER FEEL LOST AGAIN

You're seconds away from uncovering all the information you need to start your gym routine, and stick to it.

Publisher: Independent Publishing Network

www.bookisbn.org.uk

Author: Aaron Choi

Please direct all enquiries to the author.

ISBN: 978-1-80352-492-4

Printed in The United Kingdom

DISCLAIMER

Weight Loss Worldwide LTD provides education with your health and safety in mind. Having said that, everyone has their limitations. To reduce the risk of an unfortunate incident from occurring, please consult a healthcare provider for safety precautions before engaging in any workout program.

Even if you don't have any existing health problems, exercise is not without it's risks. These risks include but are not limited to: risk of injury, risk of death, overexertion, muscle strains, abnormal blood pressure and fainting. I, Aaron Choi, as well as my company, Weight Loss Worldwide LTD, disclaim any liability from the guidance given in this book.

This book will also include exercise advice only. If you are interested in learning about nutrition too, feel free to contact me via one of the methods below. I will be happy to refer you to some books and websites that I deem to be useful.

WhatsApp: +447787166065
Email: aaronchoi@weightlossworldwideltd.com
Instagram: @aaronchoi_pt
Facebook: https://www.facebook.com/weightlossworldwideltd

Chapters

Chapters

CHAPTER 1: INTRODUCTION

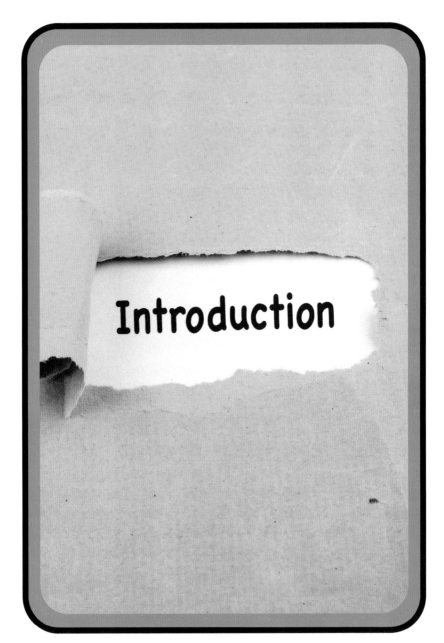

Chapter 1: Introduction

Hi there and thank you for buying my book!

My name is Aaron. I've been a personal trainer and an online fitness coach for the last five years. In this time, I've had hundreds of clients who had joined a gym for the first time and I always seem to notice the same thing when I initially talk to them; they're either anxious, uncomfortable, or terrified! This is mainly due to the fear of the unknown.

The fear of the unknown can cause you to imagine scary scenarios in your head about what might happen once you've signed up. If you too imagine these scenarios, or suffer from any of these feelings, I want you to realise that you're not alone!

I know so many people who felt the same way and, in a lot of cases, it was too overwhelming to overcome. Unfortunately that meant, for many, they never even got to start their self improvement journey.

I'm going to ask you to trust me. I've written this book to help avoid that happening to you! So, we're going to explore some of the common issues that might mentally, or physically, be preventing you from joining a gym including a lack of time, gym anxiety, a lack of confidence, worrying that people will be watching you, and more! With each of these 'barriers', I'll be finding a realistic and achievable set of solutions to prevent these issues from keeping you away from your personal goals.

The good news is that when you're given the right strategies and encouragement, those feelings soon disappear! I've seen it happen time and time again through training my clients over the years. Within a few months, or sometimes even just a few weeks, I've seen mindsets completely change. My clients begin a steady shift from dreading their gym sessions, to actively looking forward to them! How? Well, that's within the pages of this book which I now want to share with you. Because when you have that support from me, your goals are going to be within reach, not out of it!

I'm going to be sharing my experiences with you and, together, we'll explore important aspects of the gym, such as how to:

- identify the right type of exercise for you
- structure your workouts
- perform exercises correctly

So whether you're looking to join a gym, or you're already a member but feeling like you've lost your motivation, I've got you covered! I'll explain all the steps in understandable and realistic terms. When you finish reading this book, you'll have the tools you need to be at that gym consistently – and finally get that body confidence you deserve!

Are you ready?

Let's do this!

CHAPTER 2:
WHY I WANT TO HELP YOU

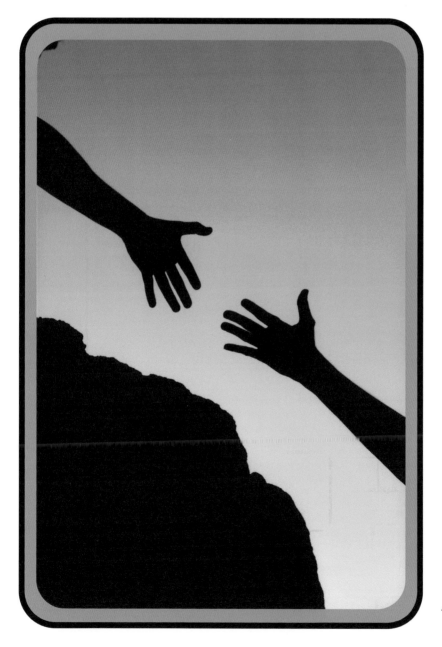

CHAPTER 2: WHY I WANT TO HELP YOU

(MY STORY!)

Before we go any further I'd like to share a little of my own story which will explain why I feel so passionate about helping you.

Let me start by saying this; I know how it feels to not be fully happy with yourself. I first wanted to join a gym when I was 16 because I had significant confidence issues. These stemmed from how I saw myself and also how I felt others saw me.

Growing up, I had severe acne and eczema all over my body. These two things made me extremely self conscious and had a serious, negative impact on how I perceived myself which then affected my self worth. On top of that, I was stick thin!

Now, I know there are many people who are underweight – and arguably more who would like to be thinner. However, when I say I was 'stick thin', I mean worryingly underweight. I was physically weak and had no additional muscle than the bare minimum to function. I felt I needed to make a change and knew I had to take control.

I decided I was going to start going to a gym and add some size to my frame. But there was a problem; I had absolutely no idea what to do! I had never even walked into a gym, let alone used the equipment. What if people laughed at me? What if I looked totally out of place, among the body Gods! What if I made a complete fool of myself?!

I felt anxious and, looking back now, probably a bit paranoid. I was so underweight, weak and unfit, I was scared that people would laugh at me, attempting to lift even the smallest weights! These thoughts soon became so convincing, they stopped me going consistently to the gym. I would go one week, then tell myself it was pointless and miss the next. This continued for some time. Sound familiar?

MY STORY

Another common theme which I was also guilty of is that when most people do join a gym, they often don't ask for help from professionals. This results in a lengthy trial and error process while they try to figure out what works and, yes... this is what happened to me! I wasted years in the gym never progressing as much as I wanted to. The result was frustration which resulted in me almost giving up, several times! I really don't want you to travel the same lengthy road I did. I have the knowledge and experience to shorten that journey so you don't experience the same disappointment and frustration I did. By reading this book, and making that commitment to yourself, you'll be provided with the right information to get your gym routine up and running. And when, not if, all goes well, you won't have wasted all that time – like I did!

Just because you might not be in a great place, physically, right now, that doesn't mean you don't have truly great potential! If someone had told me, when I was sixteeen, that I would reach the strength levels that I've now reached, there is no way that I would have believed them. I was lifting really low weights when I started, and I genuinely struggled to lift them! It was even more disheartening to look around and feel like everyone else was lifting heavier weights and making it look almost easy! But, after years of training, I'm now at a point where I'm stronger than I ever thought I could, or would, be!

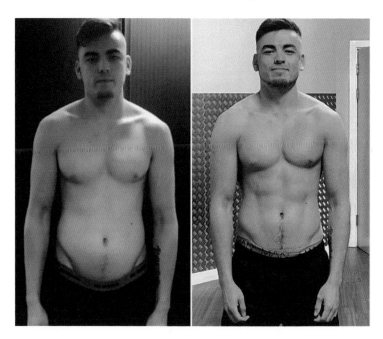

MY STORY

The beautiful thing is that I've seen the same happen with my clients, many of whom started when their self-confidence and self-esteem was truly low. But with my guidance, encouragement and their commitment, they were able to achieve truly fantastic results!

So while I can understand how easy it is to doubt yourself, and what you're capable of, please trust me that these thoughts will weaken as you watch your body strengthen. The great thing about starting at this point is you have so much more to gain. You are going to feel so proud of what you accomplish because the difference will be more noticeable to you...and all those around you!

One of the reasons I want to help you is because I know how much of an impact getting into shape can have on your life. It's been one of the main factors that helped me with my issues and become a much happier person, both inside and out. My confidence levels slowly began to increase as I started noticing changes in my shape, my strength and in the comments from family and friends. Now, I can honestly say I am the most confident I have ever been. I definitely would not have been able to say that if it hadn't been for the gym. I'd love for you to experience the same thing. It's very common for people to join a gym purely to improve their physical appearance. But, when your physical appearance starts to change, so, too, will your inner-self...you soon realise there are almost endless benefits to your commitment and determination, including:

- Increased confidence
- Increased energy levels
- Raised libido
- Improvements in your mood
- Reduced stress levels
- Better sleep quality

MY STORY

Plus a whole bunch of other cool stuff will happen!

Imagine the impact that all of these benefits will have on your life. It has happened to me - and I know the same can happen to you. So this is the time for you to start getting excited. Changes are coming your way!

The final reason that I want to help you is because now, more than ever, it's important to look after yourself. We're living in a strange time...the soils we're growing our food in are becoming less fertile so the foods we're eating are being stripped of their goodness. The water we drink has heavy metals and chemicals which damage our health and almost all the food that we buy in supermarkets contain microplastics. And that's just the physical side of things!

Mentally, people of all ages, genders and cultures are struggling more now than ever before, with weekly statistics to prove it. The level of expectation we put on ourselves due to societal pressure is huge. With social media influencing how we perceive ourselves, our world and the part we play in it, it's easy to look out at the fancy lifestyles, 'perfect' bodies and gleaming, white teeth and feel inferior, or like we're failing somehow. We naturally compare ourselves to these people which then damages our own self worth. This can then lead to us believing we're not worthy of changing, or improving. But that can't be true. You ARE worth the effort and you ARE worth improving.

And guess what? You've already taken the first step in improving yourself by buying this book. That's a great start! Now we are going to progress from this point, step by step, slowly transforming you into a fitter, healthier, more confident version of the already unique and brilliant person you are!

Let's go!

CLIENT SPOTLIGHT
YOU DON'T HAVE TO GET RID OF YOUR SOCIAL LIFE!

CHRIS Nurse London, UK

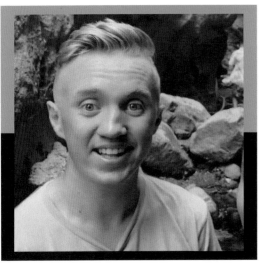

Before Chris contacted me, he wasn't feeling too happy with himself. He had gained a fair bit of body fat and wasn't in the best physical shape. He wanted to change this, but just didn't have the motivation to go to the gym and workout. He preferred to spend his spare time socialising and drinking with friends, and he made that clear when he spoke to me.

I told Chris that wasn't a problem, as I knew he could still get in good shape while maintaining his heavy social life. I built a plan that worked around this part of his life and gave him targets to hit that allowed him to progress while still being able to go out at the weekend.

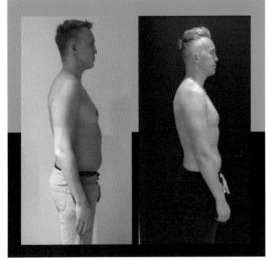

The result is that Chris lost a lot of weight, built a lot of strength, and improved his health. He did all of this while having fun at the weekend too!

Chris is proof that if you do things right, you can go out and still progress well. You don't have to eliminate everything that you enjoy from your life!

9

CHAPTER 3:
UNDERSTANDING GYM TERMS

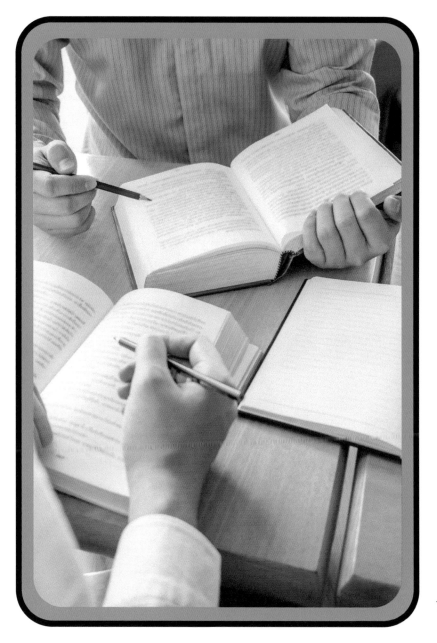

UNDERSTANDING GYM TERMS

In this section, we'll be going over the following terms:

1. Reps
2. Sets
3. TUT (Time under tension)
4. ROM (Range of motion)
5. Failure
6. DOMS (Delayed onset muscle soreness)
7. Progressive overload
8. PB (Personal best)
9. Free Weights
10. Supersets
11. Dropsets
12. Spotter
13. HIIT
14. Isolation exercises
15. Compound exercises
16. Deload week
17. Rest periods
18. Hypertrophy
19. Volume
20. Dynamic Stretching
21. Static Stretching

UNDERSTANDING GYM TERMS

For the stage that most of you are at, it is likely that you will not understand the language that people who go to the gym talk in. But don't worry, I've got you covered. Here's a list of the most used phrases that people use when they talk about the gym. Give these terms a read, and you'll sound like a pro in no time!

1. <u>Reps</u>

This is a commonly used gym term and is simply short for repetitions. Repetitions are the number of times you lift a weight fully up and down before dropping it. For instance, if you did 10 reps of bicep curls, you would have curled that weight up and down 10 times.

If you want to predominantly build strength, typically, you want to do a lower amount of reps with a heavier weight. For example, doing between 5 and 10 reps. Whereas if you want to predominantly build more endurance, you should perform a higher amount of reps with a lighter weight. For example, 15 to 20 reps.

When you pick a rep range, it's important to know that you need to fail in that rep range. For instance, let's say that you do 5 to 10 reps of squats. This is an example of how you should roughly feel:

Reps 1-5: it's not feeling too bad
Rep 6: it's starting to get a bit hard now
Rep 7: ok this is quite painful now
Rep 8: I don't think that I can keep going
Rep 9 or 10: Failure

UNDERSTANDING GYM TERMS

Your sets will not look exactly like this. In fact, you can fail at rep 5 in this rep range, and this wouldn't be a problem. The point is that you need to fail in this range. When you do, over the next few weeks you need to keep trying to increase the reps until you're at the top of the rep range. When you are, then you increase the weight and drop to the bottom of the rep range again. Then you keep this process going.

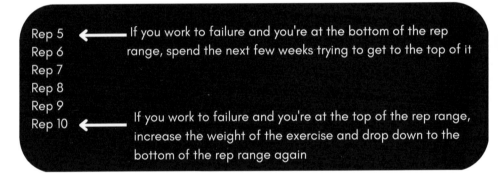

Rep 5 ⟵——— If you work to failure and you're at the bottom of the rep
Rep 6   range, spend the next few weeks trying to get to the top of it
Rep 7
Rep 8
Rep 9
Rep 10 ⟵   If you work to failure and you're at the top of the rep range,
                     increase the weight of the exercise and drop down to the
                     bottom of the rep range again

It's also important to note that if you don't fail in your rep range, you either have not worked hard enough or haven't picked the right weight. So, when I say "do 5-10 reps", you shouldn't casually just do that number of reps before dropping the weight. If that is the case, then one or both of those situations are happening!

In the vast majority of cases, I would recommend incorporating both higher reps and lower rep ranges into your workouts. Both amounts of reps can result in muscle growth, and therefore, both are good at changing your body.

UNDERSTANDING GYM TERMS

2. Sets

A set simply refers to a collection of reps. For instance, imagine that you did 10 reps of bicep curls. After that, if you proceeded to drop the weight and rest a minute before doing the same thing again, you would have performed 2 sets of 10 reps.

Typically, I would recommend doing 2-4 sets per exercise per session in the gym. More is definitely not better though, as it's diminishing returns with every extra set you do. So, I would recommend going for high quality sets rather than prioritising quantity.

3. TUT (Time under tension)

This refers to the amount of time your muscles are working during a set. Putting your muscles under tension for too long is extremely important if you want to build strength and muscle. Typically speaking with each exercise, you should aim for:
- 3 seconds on the lengthening phase
- an optional 1 second pause
- 1 second on the shortening phase
- an optional 1 second pause

As you can see, each rep should last 4-6 seconds. However, the vast majority of gym goers will rush through their reps, therefore limiting the time under tension. This will in turn hinder their results. Rushing reps is one reason why people never progress how they want to in a gym! So, remember, quicker is not better.

UNDERSTANDING GYM TERMS

4. ROM (Range of motion)

The range of motion of an exercise refers to the distance that you move a weight during each rep. The larger the range of motion, the more muscle fibres you will work, and in turn the better your results will be. Lots of people will lift with their ego and limit the range of motion to make the exercise easier. This will in turn mean that you can lift more weight. However, this is a bad idea. You will almost always achieve better results using a full range of motion, even if you lift less weight. So, aim for high levels of ROM!

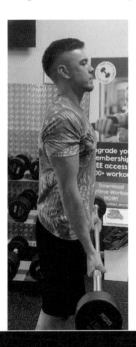 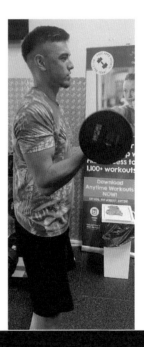

This exercise is a bicep curl, where you are meant to curl the weight up to your upper chest. After this, you're meant to lower the weight until your arms are straight at the bottom. As you can see in these pictures, I have done both of these things. Therefore, the range of motion is very good.

UNDERSTANDING GYM TERMS

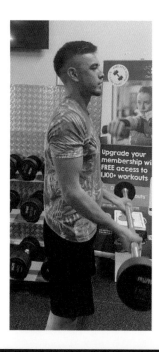 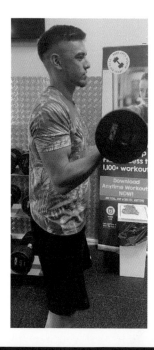

These are a different set of photos. Even though I am curling the weight up to my upper chest height in the second photo, I'm not fully straightening my arms in the first one. Therefore, the range of motion isn't as good as it should be.

UNDERSTANDING GYM TERMS

5. Failure

This might sound like something that you don't want to come across, but it's crucial that you do if you want to progress. When you work close to failure, it means that you keep going until you almost cannot lift that weight anymore. This should be the goal for you as when you push your muscles and make them work hard, they're far more likely to change. While I don't recommend going to absolute failure all the time, I would recommend working to at least a 7 or 8/10 in terms of difficulty in the vast majority of your sets.

If you finish a set and the set was not a struggle, you probably haven't challenged your muscles enough to warrant them changing. So, make sure that you push yourself!

6. DOMS (Delayed Onset Muscle Soreness)

This is the pain that you may feel in the next few days after you finish a workout, and stems from your muscles being damaged. This is not something to be concerned about. At the end of the day, if your muscles are being damaged then they are being challenged. And if they are being challenged, then they're more likely to change!

You'll normally get bad DOMS in the first few weeks or months of lifting, or if you suddenly incorporate a different stimulus, such as a new exercise. However, it is normal for the feelings to get less and less severe over time anyway. This is also nothing to be concerned about, as high levels of DOMS does not equate to high levels of muscle growth. In truth, you can build muscle and progress without experiencing much DOMS at all. So, if you finish a workout and you're not sore, don't panic!

UNDERSTANDING GYM TERMS

7. Progressive Overload

Progressive overload basically refers to your gym work gradually getting harder over time. This can be accomplished in multiple ways, such as:
- increasing the weight
- increasing the range of motion
- increasing the number of reps that you do
- increasing the time under tension
- improving the overall form
- doing more total sets (up to a point)

All of these will result in your muscles being put under more stress. And like we have just spoken about; your body will be more likely to change when it's put under more stress. While you don't need to make the exercises that you're doing harder every single session, you should aim to do this as frequently as possible. If you don't give your body a reason to want to change, then it will not! If your goal is to trim down, build strength and/or build muscle, progressive overload is something you need to prioritise!

8. PB (Personal best)

When someone says that they have just hit a PB, it means that they have hit a new personal best. This could involve them lifting a certain weight for more reps than they did before, lifting more weight than they did before, or any other method that would make things harder. Whatever the scenario, it's important to hit PB's as much as possible. Because, you're more likely to force your body to change if the stimulus gets harder. PB's are also a great way to build your confidence too, which will spark your motivation to keep your training going!

UNDERSTANDING GYM TERMS

9. Free weights

Free weights are weights you lift that are not attached to a particular set of equipment. These include:
- Dumbbells
- Kettlebells
- Barbells

Although I wouldn't necessarily say that free weights always lead to better results than machines, they tend to be more effective most of the time. They are also generally harder to lift as they require more coordination, technique, and stability. Therefore, I recommend that you incorporate some of the equipment that I've mentioned above in your training program.

This doesn't have to be straight away though. It's much easier to use these pieces of equipment incorrectly, especially as a beginner, because you have limited knowledge and experience at this point. But as a beginner, you can progress fine without using them too much. Initially, I would recommend you use more machines, and then scale up to doing more free weight exercises over time while your confidence and skill set builds.

Because of the potential complexity of the lifts involving these pieces of equipment, it's common for beginners to avoid them altogether due to the fear of them performing them wrong in front of people. This is especially the case for any exercise that involves using barbells in the free weights area. Whereas your possible fears and anxiety levels will be much lower when you use machines. This means that you're more likely to get these exercises done instead!

UNDERSTANDING GYM TERMS

10. Supersets

A superset involves you performing two exercises back-to-back with no rest in between. For example, a set of squats followed by a set of push ups.

These can be useful to perform as they limit the amount of time that you must spend in the gym to finish your workout. The downside is that because you don't rest as long, they can make your muscles and your whole body more tired. Therefore, the amount you perform them partially depends on your level of fitness. They are also not essential to do in general.

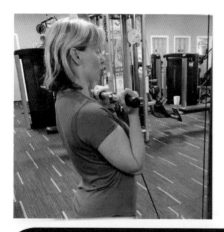 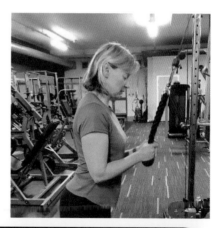

These exercises show a classic example of a superset. The first exercise is a cable bicep curl, and the second exercise is a tricep pushdown. These two exercises go great together, as they work the upper part of your arm in a short amount of time!

UNDERSTANDING GYM TERMS

11. Dropsets

Drop Sets involve you doing multiple sets of one exercise back-to-back, dropping the weight each time you get to the point of near failure. For example, this could involve you doing:

- 10 reps of a bicep curl with a 20kg bar
- 9 reps of a bicep curl with a 15kg bar
- 6 reps of a bicep curl with a 10kg bar

You would perform all these sets one after another, with no rest in between.

Drop sets are an effective way to work hard and can lead to decent muscle and strength gains. However, they can be quite difficult so are not something that beginners normally do. I wouldn't not recommend doing them. But at the same time, they aren't essential to do. As a beginner with limited knowledge and experience, it might also be possible that you cheat your way through certain sets when it gets tough. This is to make the lifting easier. If this is the case, you may not gain all the benefits of the drop set while increasing the risk of an injury occurring.

UNDERSTANDING GYM TERMS

12. Spotter

A spotter is someone who assists you or stands by you during an exercise. This is mainly to make sure that you perform the exercise correctly and safely. The most common exercise to have a spotter is during a bench press. This involves someone standing behind you just in case you can't lift the weight.

Having a spotter can be a great way to work harder during a set. It also increases your confidence during it, as you know someone can help you if you struggle!

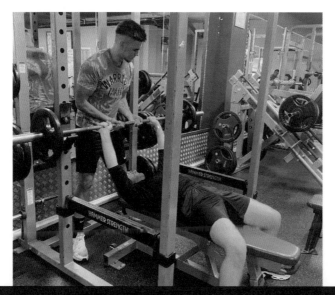

In this picture, I'm being a spotter for my friend while he bench presses. Me being behind him makes him feel more comfortable during the set.

UNDERSTANDING GYM TERMS

13. HIIT

HIIT stands for High Intensity Interval Training, which is a form of cardiovascular exercise that you can do. This training involves periods of high intensity work followed by brief low intensity periods, or full-on rest periods. You then repeat this for a certain amount of time. A simple example is sprinting for 15 seconds, and then doing a slow walk for 30 seconds, which you would then repeat 10 times.

Performing HIIT workouts can be great if you're time strapped, as they typically don't last too long. They're also pretty good at improving your levels of fitness. The main downside, however, is that you may not perform exercises correctly when you get tired. And if this is the case, you can increase your risk of injury. I would therefore recommend limiting your HIIT workouts if you have a low level of fitness, experience and/or knowledge. Regardless though, just like supersets and drop sets, they are not essential to include in your workout routine in the first place.

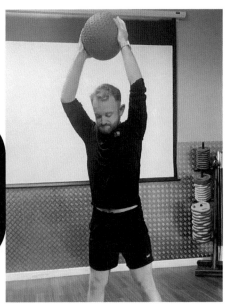

In this picture, ball slams are being performed. This is a classic exercise that's performed in a HIIT workout. This exercise would be performed alongside other exercises, with periods of rest in between.

UNDERSTANDING GYM TERMS

14. Isolation Exercises

An isolation exercise involves you lifting a weight through just one joint. For example, a bicep curl. In this case, the weight moves solely through your elbow joint, and nothing else.

Isolation exercises are great at targeting specific weak areas. They are also quite simple to perform as these exercises don't involve as much concentration as some of the other exercises you can do at the gym.

The downside of these exercises is that because you only have one joint contributing to the move, you can't lift a huge amount of weight. This isn't a massive problem, as isolation exercises are still great to perform. However, typically speaking your body will change more if the intensity of the lift is higher, and lifting heavier weights is a great way to make the lift more intense.

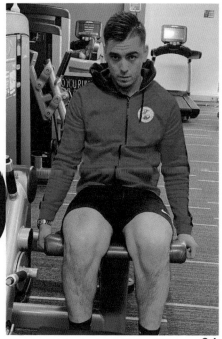

In this picture, leg extensions are being performed. This is an isolation exercise, as the only joint involved is your knee joint.

UNDERSTANDING GYM TERMS

15. Compound Exercises

Compound exercises involve you lifting weight through more than one joint. For example, a squat. This involves you moving weight through your hips and knees at the same time.

The great thing about compound moves is that because you work multiple joints, you work multiple muscles too. When this is the case, you can lift more weight as you have more parts of your body contributing to the lift. When you lift more weight, typically speaking you can build more strength and muscle. Therefore, prioritising compound lifts should be a priority for you if you want to change your body!

The downside of compound exercises is that they are typically harder to perform. This is because you must pay attention to more aspects of these lifts. If you're a beginner, you might find these more confusing to learn than the isolation exercises. However, you should still perform lots of these, as these will change your body more than isolation exercises!

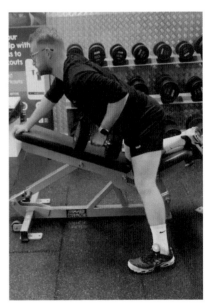

In this picture, a one arm dumbbell row is being performed. This is a compound exercise, as you can move weight through your elbow and your shoulder joint.

UNDERSTANDING GYM TERMS

16. Deload week

A deload week is a scheduled week where you reduce the intensity and/or the amount of work you do. For example, just doing some walking or stretching. Sometimes it can also involve you just taking a complete break from the gym altogether.

Although you might think that taking things easy for a week will interfere with your progress, it often results in the opposite effect. Resting your muscles and your central nervous system gives both a chance to recover. When this happens, you will find that you'll feel fresher and stronger going into the next week. So, although it isn't necessary to take deload weeks, I would recommend taking one every few months for this reason.

17. Rest periods

Rest periods are the periods of time in between your working sets. For example, let's say you do 10 reps of bicep curls, and then rest for a minute before going again. Your rest period in this case would be 60 seconds. The amount of time that you should rest, depends on a couple of factors, predominantly:

1) The intensity at which you're working
If you're working at a higher intensity, you will need longer rest periods
Whereas if the intensity is quite low, then you can afford to jump into the next set a little bit quicker.

2) The amount of weight that you're lifting
Typically speaking, the heavier you lift the more you'll need to rest. Whereas lighter weights normally involve shorter rest periods.

UNDERSTANDING GYM TERMS

3) The type of exercise that you're doing

If you're doing a compound exercise, then this will require more energy from your body. In this case, you will need to rest a little longer. On the other hand, isolation movements don't require as much energy therefore don't require long rest periods.

Because of these three variables, it's hard to give you an exact amount of time you should rest between each set. This is especially the case when you consider individual differences between us, such as our level of fitness level and any physical problems that we may have. Typically though, this is what I would recommend:

Heavy compound movements: 2-5 minutes
Lighter Isolation movements: 1-2 minutes

18. Hypertrophy

Hypertrophy is just another term for muscle gain. If the muscles on your body seem larger or harder, then the process of hypertrophy has taken place.

UNDERSTANDING GYM TERMS

19. Volume

Volume refers to the amount of work that you do in the gym. You can increase volume by either increasing the number of reps that you do, or the number of sets you do. Both will increase the total amount of work you have to do for your muscle groups per week.

The amount of volume you need per muscle per week can vary. Some people who have good genetics can get away with incorporating less volume and can still experience great results. Your diet also matters. If you're trying to put on muscle but aren't consuming enough calories, then too much volume throughout your week can even be detrimental in some cases. Another factor is also the intensity at which you train. If you work harder in certain sets, then you can afford to get away with incorporating less total volume throughout your week, as the stimulus may still be strong enough to drive hypertrophy.

As a typical rule of thumb though, I would say that the ideal volume range for most muscles for most people is around 10-20 total sets per week. If you go over this amount, it is diminishing returns and won't help you as much as you think. However, if you're under 10 total sets per muscle per week, then your volume may not be high enough to drive hypertrophy. 10-20 total sets is a bit of a sweet spot amongst most people.

UNDERSTANDING GYM TERMS

20. Dynamic Stretching

Dynamic stretching involves stretching while moving. They're controlled movements that prepare your muscles to perform safely. For that reason, dynamic stretching is best performed before a workout. This will increase your range of motion through certain joints, and warm up the joint and its surrounding muscles.

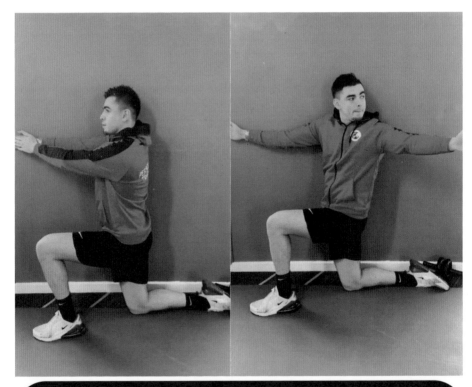

The pictures above show a type of thoracic extension. This involves mobilising the back while moving. Therefore, it's an example of a dynamic stretch.

UNDERSTANDING GYM TERMS

21. Static Stretching

Static stretching involves you moving a muscle as far as it can go without any strong pain, and then holding it in that position for a certain amount of time (typically around 45 seconds.) As this doesn't involve moving, it has different benefits compared to dynamic stretching. In fact, doing static stretching at the beginning of a workout may even negatively impact your workout.

Static stretching should be performed at the end of your workouts. Doing so can help reduce muscle stiffness and reduce the risk of injury.

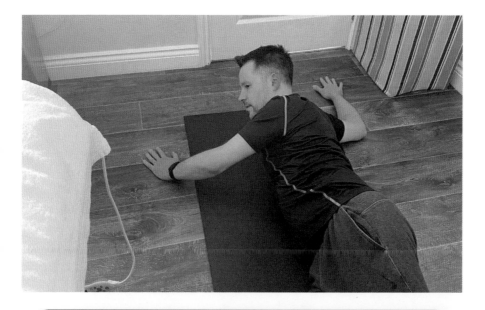

The picture above shows a type of chest stretch. This particular person is stretching his chest without moving. Therefore, this is an example of a static stretch.

JENNY Midwife London, UK

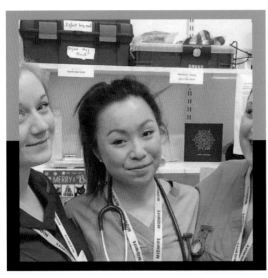

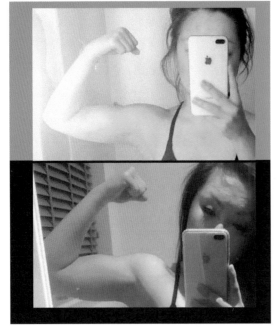

Although Jenny had been a member of a gym for a while before she reached out to me, she didn't go all that often. This was because she lacked the drive to do so. She knew she would benefit from going more, but she just didn't have the motivation to!

The thing is, lacking motivation is a problem that can easily be fixed by adding some accountability. And this is what I gave Jenny. I put a plan in place for her and checked up on her a couple of times a week to make sure that she stayed on track. Because of this, she stayed consistent with what she had to do as she didn't want to let me down.

Jenny built up a lot of muscle and strength during our time working together. This made her proud of herself which only fuelled her willingness to keep the process going.

So if you lack motivation, this honestly isn't that big of a problem. It's just up to you to reach out for help to start your journey in the first place.

CHAPTER 4:
CHOOSING THE RIGHT TYPE OF EXERCISE FOR YOU

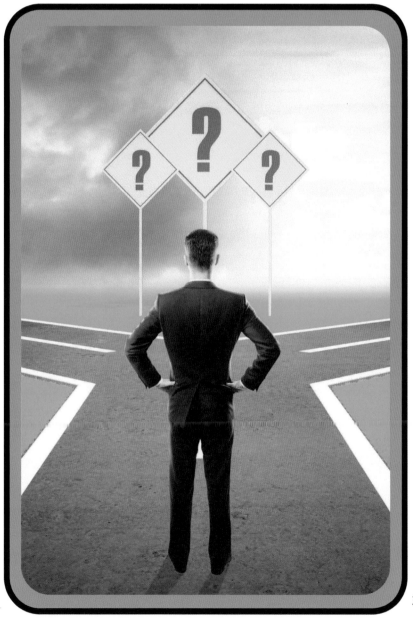

CHOOSING THE RIGHT TYPE OF EXERCISE FOR YOU

As you can probably guess, there's not a one size fits all approach when it comes to the gym. This is partly because we all have a different goal, and this dictates what type of training we should do. And this is what we're going to cover in this section. If you haven't quite worked out your goal yet, don't worry. I've highlighted 8 main goals below for you to have a look at, and what type(s) of training you should do to hit each of them. Before you move on to the next section, make sure you firmly decide on what goal you would like to achieve!

1. Improving your general health and fitness

If you don't care about changing how you look too much, or if progressing in the gym isn't a huge priority for you right now, this could be a good goal for you to work towards.

Doing a little bit of everything in the gym will improve most key aspects of fitness and ,therefore, make you fairly well-rounded. If this sounds good to you, I recommend doing a little bit of cardio, weight training, and mobility work. If you do this, you will build up some experience in each area, so you can become more familiar with how to partake in multiple types of training.

However, the downside of this approach is that because you incorporate a few different types of training throughout your week, you will probably never excel at any aspect of the gym. This doesn't mean you can't change your goal at a later date though.

CHOOSING THE RIGHT TYPE OF EXERCISE FOR YOU

2. Improving your flexibility and mobility

As you can probably guess, if you want to improve your flexibility and mobility, then stretching should be the biggest part of your gym routine. You can do two main types of flexibility work: dynamic and static. Both have numerous benefits, such as improving the range of motion in your joints and reducing your risk of injuries. Doing mobility work can also be good for your mental health due to its ability to release tension and help you feel more relaxed after!

It's also important to note that weight training can be good at improving your mobility, when it is performed through a full range of motion. Therefore, if this is your goal, I would predominantly do mobility work, with a little bit of weight training on the side.

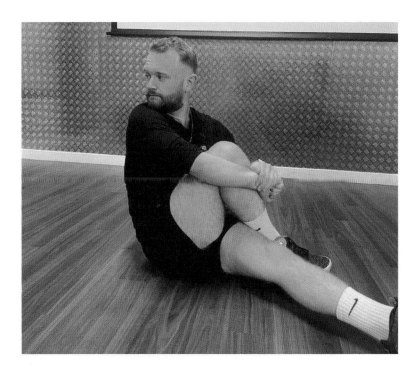

CHOOSING THE RIGHT TYPE OF EXERCISE FOR YOU

3. Improving your cardiovascular fitness

If you want to improve your cardiovascular fitness, then doing predominantly cardio is the way to go. There are several different types of cardio you can do in the gym. On the gym floors of most gyms, you will find treadmills, rowing machines, cross trainers, and bicycles. There is also the option of doing a bodyweight routine such as a HIIT workout. All these options can greatly improve your cardio ability.

If you want to get better at a certain type of cardio, I would mainly stick to that. This is because specificity is crucial when it comes to getting better in the gym. For instance, if you want to train to run a half marathon, you should mainly stick to the treadmill. However, if you don't want to get better at a certain type of cardio then I would just do what you enjoy the most. This is because you're more likely to stick with your training long term. If I tell someone who hates running to run on the treadmill, chances are they will not last long!

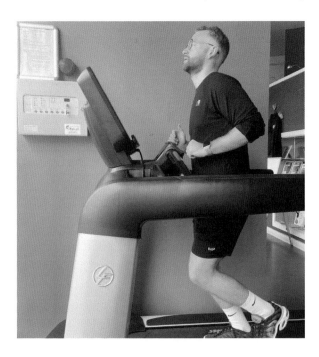

CHOOSING THE RIGHT TYPE OF EXERCISE FOR YOU

4. Building muscle and strength

You guessed it. If this is your goal, weight training is where it's at! Weight training provides the stimulus for muscle growth. Therefore, most of your training should be purely lifting weights.

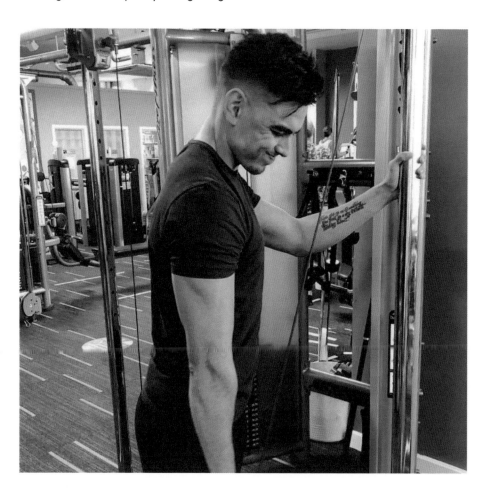

CHOOSING THE RIGHT TYPE OF EXERCISE FOR YOU

5. Losing weight

Now, this is something that might surprise you. Contrary to popular belief, cardio is not the best way to lose weight! This is because, health benefits aside, all cardio does is burn calories. You might say that sounds great, but the problem is that it's much easier to consume calories than to burn them. For instance, eating two doughnuts may lead to you taking in about 500 calories. And realistically, it may only take a couple of minutes to eat them. Whereas if you tried to burn 500 calories, that would take you close to an hour! Therefore, if you want to lose weight, controlling what you eat is the main priority.

On top of that, weight training can make the process of losing weight a lot easier. This is because your metabolism speeds up when you lift weights and build muscle. If this happens, your body is going to be in a much better state to burn more calories at rest. This will in turn lead to it being easier to stay lean in the long run! So, if losing weight is your main goal, then you need to follow a solid weight training plan. And if you want, throw in a little bit of cardio training to burn some excess calories on the side. However, please make sure that you never replace your weight training with cardio!

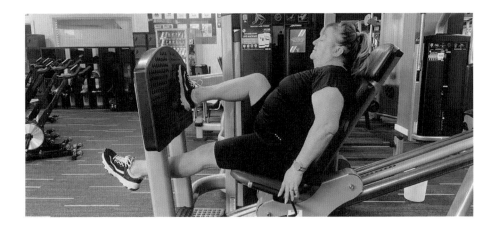

CHOOSING THE RIGHT TYPE OF EXERCISE FOR YOU

6. Toning up

'Toning' up is a common fitness goal. However, I need to make something clear. 'Toning' up isn't a thing! There's no physical way to 'tone' or 'shape' a muscle. You can only build it.

Typically, when people say they want to 'tone' up, they want to lose weight and build muscle at the same time. If this is the case, then weight training should be your priority. This is because weight training not only promotes muscle growth, but in turn, it can also speed up your metabolism making losing weight a lot easier! Like with losing weight, throwing in a little bit of cardio can help burn some extra calories, but isn't going to make as strong of a difference as weight training will. So, if your goal is to 'tone' up, then make sure you lift a lot of weights!

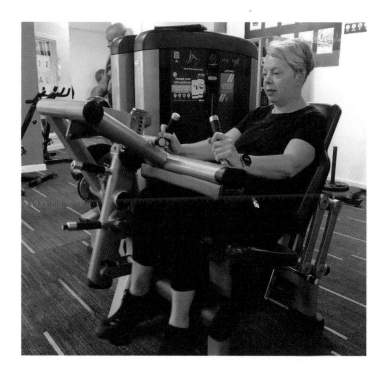

CHOOSING THE RIGHT TYPE OF EXERCISE FOR YOU

7. Rehab

If your goal is to rehab an injury of some sort, the best move would be to consult a physiotherapist. Getting a part of your body back to normal can be a long and specific process and is not something you can typically figure out on your own. Especially as a beginner!

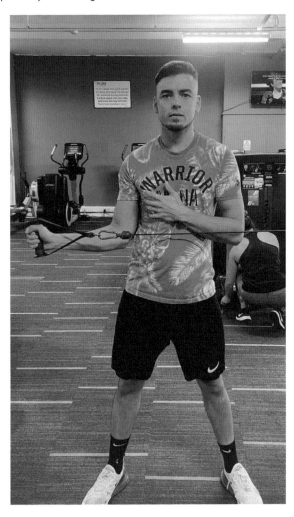

CHOOSING THE RIGHT TYPE OF EXERCISE FOR YOU

8. Staying healthy at an older age

If you're at an older age and reading this, I think it's terrific that you're wanting to improve your health and overall quality of life! The first thing that I want to say is that just because it normally gets slightly harder to get in shape when you're older, doesn't mean that it's not do-able! In fact, I've had plenty of clients in their 50's and 60's achieve great results!

If you're in this boat then your goal should be to counteract three big negative effects of aging: having your metabolism slow down, losing mobility, and losing muscle. And there there's one thing that you can do to counteract all three at the same time: lift weights! As previously mentioned, lifting weights can speed up your metabolism as well as improve your mobility and ability to build muscle. Therefore, if you're an older individual, then weight training should be your number one priority!

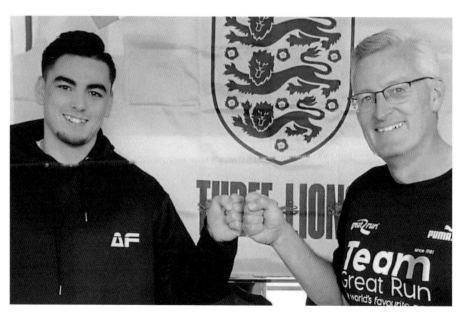

CLIENT SPOTLIGHT
PERSONALISED PROGRAMS ALWAYS WIN!

WILL Cardiac Physiologist London, UK

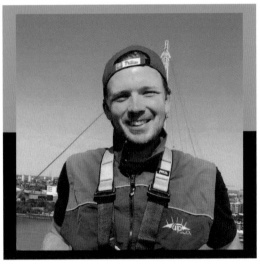

Will is a close friend of mine who I have known for many years. And while he has always been in decent shape, he knew he could be doing better. At this point, Will mainly followed generic workout plans that you can find for free online. And his results weren't as he wanted.

After he reached out to me, I made him a personalised plan that was tailored perfectly to him. He built up an insane amount of muscle and strength very quickly, to the point where he genuinely ended up making more progress in a few months than he did in the last few years combined!

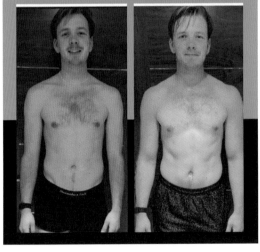

I understand the temptation to not invest in yourself, as it can be a bit of an investment. But if you do go ahead with it, you will be very satisfied with the results. Plus, your quality of life will go tremendously. So if getting in shape means a lot to you, this is an option that you should definitely consider.

41

CHAPTER 5:
UNDERSTANDING SPEED OF PROGRESS

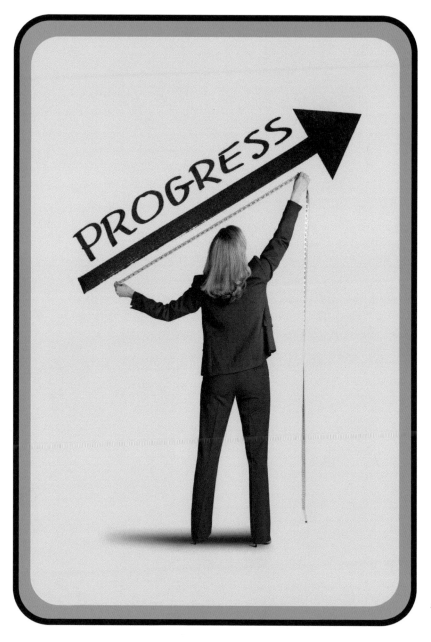

UNDERSTANDING SPEED OF PROGRESS

1. Improving your fitness

You can improve your fitness by improving your cardiovascular ability, your strength levels, and/or your mobility.

The good news is that your fitness levels are the first thing to improve. In fact, if you do things right, you can see improvements in your fitness pretty quickly, especially as a beginner! This is because the gym is a fresh, novel stimulus for your body. As a result, you can see fitness improvements quicker than someone who has much more experience than you. So, if all goes well, in just 3-4 months you can expect to notice some incredible differences in your fitness levels!

The bad news is that after a period of abstinence for whatever reason, fitness is the first thing you lose as well. It's common to lose some strength after not lifting weights for a couple of weeks! However, this is not something to be worried about. This is because it's actually quite straightforward to regain what you once had. It's just difficult to gain the strength in the first place! So, even if you do notice your levels of fitness go down after a couple of weeks off, it won't take you that much time at all to get back to where you were.

UNDERSTANDING SPEED OF PROGRESS

2. Altering your body composition

Altering your body composition is typically a slower process than building your levels of fitness. The two ways of changing how your body looks are dropping body fat, and building muscle. The rate of progress between the two is also quite different.

The rate at which you can drop body fat is largely dictated by how much you initially weigh in the first place. Typically, you can drop weight quicker if you start off at a higher body fat percentage. Regardless of how you look though, it's very possible to drop a certain amount of body fat every week. A good weight loss range is between 0.5lbs to 1.5lbs a week for the average person. So, think about how much weight you might want to lose, and then do the math on how long it might take you to get there.

There might also be some weeks where you do everything right, but still don't drop any weight. This isn't something to be alarmed about, as it doesn't mean that you will not drop any weight in the weeks after. It might also be possible that you've temporarily gained a bit of water weight, which could've counteracted the body fat that you've lost. This can stem from eating a few too many carbs, eating too much salt, your time of the month as a woman, and many more things. So, if you feel like you've been on track and your weight suddenly shoots up, don't panic. Because, unless you've been eating too many calories, it's unlikely that you've gained actual body fat. The most likely answer is that you might be carrying some extra water weight. If this is the case, then your weight should drop straight back down to normal within the next week.

UNDERSTANDING SPEED OF PROGRESS

So, although people of a larger size can drop body fat more quickly, it's possible for most people to drop body fat pretty consistently. And if you do drop weight most weeks, this will really add up. It's very possible to lose a stone in just a couple of months! You just have to make sure that you're doing everything that you should be doing, as consistently as possible.

I previously mentioned that a good weight loss range is between 0.5lbs to 1.5lbs a week. However, with muscle growth, it takes far longer to gain the equivalent in muscle mass. The good news though is that if you're a beginner, you can build muscle far quicker than people who are in better shape than you. You can also build muscle quicker than people with more experience than you, and who know more than you! This is again because the gym will be a fresh, novel stimulus for your body. As a result, your body will adapt and change more quickly. If you're a guy and you're just starting, you can build a couple of pounds of muscle most months for your first year. As a woman, you will typically build a little less than that even if you do everything right. This is because women can't build as much muscle as men, mainly due to the fact their levels of testosterone are so much lower. One thing to remember is that for every year that you lift weights, your ability to build muscle goes down and down. In years 2-3, you will probably only be able to build a maximum of half of what you built in year 1. The number will most likely be less than that though. So, the likelihood is if you're reading this right now you're in a good spot. Enjoy the quick muscle growth while you can!

UNDERSTANDING SPEED OF PROGRESS

Now, you have an idea of how long it may take you to hit your goals. Despite outlining these time frames though, I need to make something clear. These are only rough! In fact, it's actually quite hard to give time frames. This is because your speed of progress is dependent on so many things. Here are some of the top factors that will decide how quickly you may or may not progress:

1. Genetics

Unfortunately, fitness isn't fair. Sure, hard work is very important. But regardless of how hard you work, it's likely that you'll meet people who seem to progress more than you when they actually do less. If this is the case, they will have superior genetics to you. This isn't something to be too disappointed about, as everyone still has good potential to do well! Genetics just mean that some people will have a much easier time progressing and can afford to make more mistakes.

In terms of weight loss, some people will naturally have a faster metabolism than others. This means that they will find it quite easy to lose weight. In terms of muscle building, some people will have the potential to build more muscle and at a quicker rate. In fact, some people are just naturally muscular without even doing too much!

But the point remains, don't become disheartened if your genetics aren't great. When I started my muscle building journey, I was underweight for a girl. And I've still done alright for myself!

UNDERSTANDING SPEED OF PROGRESS

2. Your social life

If you're someone who has a big social life, events will likely interfere with your ability to be consistent, and therefore, your ability to make progress. The solution isn't to completely remove socialising altogether, as that's not a sustainable approach. It's about trying to enjoy yourself while limiting the damage that you do, such as limiting the amount of alcohol you drink on a night out. It's also about trying to be as consistent as possible around your social occasions, so you can then kick back and enjoy yourself without feeling too guilty.

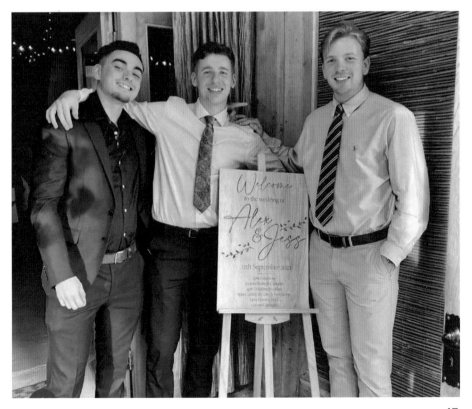

UNDERSTANDING SPEED OF PROGRESS

3. Willingness to get extra support

No matter how much experience or knowledge you have, you will always do better with someone in your corner. So, getting an online coach or a personal trainer can massively speed up your progress. This isn't just because you gain more knowledge, but it's because that person will keep you accountable. When this is the case, you're more likely to be consistent and therefore progress quicker. Without accountability, it's easy to make excuses and miss certain gym workouts when you're not in the mood to go. I personally progressed the quickest when I got a personal trainer myself, for this reason.

From my own experience, I find that women are much better at reaching out for help than men. Although I'm not entirely sure why this is the case, I feel it's probably because us men have more of an ego. Because of this, we may not reach out for help because we 'feel' like we can do it ourselves. But if you are a guy reading this, please try to not be too narrow minded! Getting a coach or a PT will honestly make such a difference, as long as you choose the right person.

UNDERSTANDING SPEED OF PROGRESS

4. Motivation dips

I feel the majority of people view motivation the wrong way. I've heard from dozens of people that they would like to join a gym, but they can't because they're not currently motivated. If this is you, I'd like you to remember one thing: motivation doesn't come and stay, motivation is just a temporary feeling! So even if you do suddenly feel that wave of motivation which does lead to you joining a gym, that feeling is just going to go away at some point anyway. Therefore, motivation is not something you can rely on to stay consistent in the long run.

If you do find that your motivation levels dip from time to time, this is normal. Almost every person will experience this. Some days will naturally just feel harder to get through than others. The good news is that there are certain things that you can do to maintain your consistency in these tougher times, thus maintaining your rate of progress. This will be covered in the 'Overcoming Your Issues' section of this book.

CHAPTER 6:
TRACKING YOUR PROGRESS

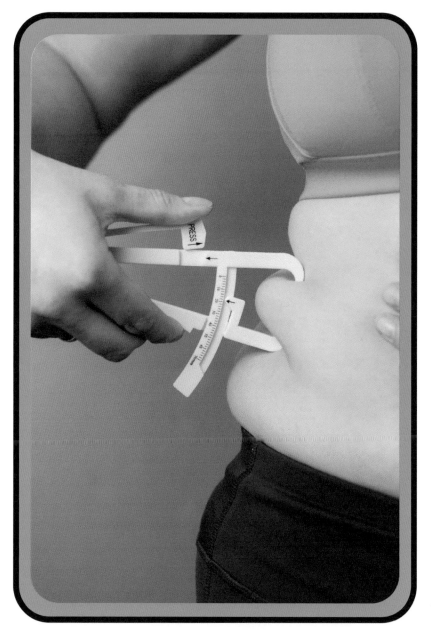

TRACKING YOUR PROGRESS

By now, you should know what goal you want to work towards, what type of training you must do to get there, and how long this might take you. Now, let's dive into ways to track your progress. I would recommend a few different methods.

1. Improving your fitness

Tracking your fitness progress is pretty straight forward.

If your goal is to improve your stamina then track how far, how fast, or long you can do a certain activity for, and then try to beat it. For example, let's say you can run on a treadmill at 8km/h for 10 minutes before having to stop. Make sure you record that. Then the next time you go in, you can either try to run at a faster speed or try to run for longer. If you've done one or both things, then you've made progress.

Tracking your flexibility and mobility is a little bit trickier to accomplish. What you are effectively trying to do is to increase your range of motion through a certain joint. Tape measures can be useful to track the differences in your range of motion. It's uncommon to see people bring these to gyms though. If your goal is to get more mobile, I would recommend doing as much mobility work as you can, and occasionally measuring your range of motion during certain moves at home. You might be able to tell by eye if your range of motion is increasing anyway, but actually measuring the changes will be a more reliable way to track progress.

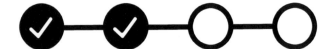

TRACKING YOUR PROGRESS

Now let's get onto how to track your strength levels changing. You can improve your strength levels in a few ways. The three easiest ways to track your strength changes are as follows:

- Increasing the weight that you lift
- Increasing the number of reps that you do
- Increasing the number of sets that you do (up to a point)

If you do these 3 things over time, then your strength levels will increase. But to know if these things are happening, it's important to be as detailed as possible when tracking what you do. You don't necessarily have to track your range of motion, technique, or any pauses, as this is a little more complicated to do. However, I would recommend that you always write down the exercise that you do, the number of sets that you do, and the weight and reps in each set. It might look something like this:

Exercise	Set	Reps	Weight (kg)
	1	10	15
Hip Thrust	2	10	15

Looking at this table, you can get an idea of what you need to do next time you're in a gym. You basically either have to aim for more than 10 reps with a 15 kg weight, or stick at 10 reps and lift a heavier weight.

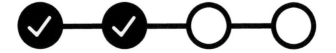

TRACKING YOUR PROGRESS

Now, you should hopefully realise that it's imperative that you track your numbers throughout your journey. Many people don't, and this is why they never progress. If you want to get stronger, but can't remember how much weight you lifted during an exercise the week before, then how on earth are you meant to know what to aim for the following week? So please try to be as consistent with your tracking as possible, so you can move in the right direction. If you don't, then progressive overload is going to be too hard to achieve.

1. Altering your body composition

When it comes to weight loss and muscle gain, I would recommend four main methods of tracking your progress.

1) Weighing yourself

Although this might seem like the best way to track your weight loss, it's often not the most reliable way to do so. As previously discussed, your body weight can and will fluctuate a lot anyway. This is mainly down to the volume of food in your stomach, or water retention. Therefore, you must not just judge your progress via the scales. It's possible to have a good week but also gain a bit of water weight. If this is the case, then your total body weight might go up. This can then really mess with your head and get you down, even though it's not something to be concerned about. Therefore, you need to track your progress in at least one more way too for more reliable judgements.

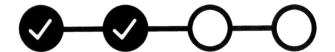

TRACKING YOUR PROGRESS

Another problem with weighing yourself is that it's possible to drop body fat and gain muscle at the same time. Although you can typically drop body fat quicker than you can gain muscle, overtime your weight could somewhat still even out. If this is the case, you will think that you haven't made any progress when you actually have.

2) Noticing how your clothes fit

If your clothes, feel a little looser then this can be a good sign that you've dropped some body fat. On the other side of the spectrum, if you're looking to build muscle then hopefully your clothes will feel tighter over time.

3) Taking Measurements

Although measurements can sometimes be misleading too, more often than not they are a fantastic way to track your progress.

The areas that I would measure would be your triceps, biceps, shoulders, chest, hips, waist, and thighs. When you measure yourself, make sure that you measure the part of your body at its thickest possible point. This is the easiest point to go back to when you remeasure yourself in the future, leading to higher levels of accuracy. Also make sure that the tape is tight, but not overly suffocating. If you're looking to drop body fat, you will be aiming for the size in all areas to go down. If you're looking to build muscle, you want all of those areas to increase in size except for your waist. I would recommend taking measurements every month.

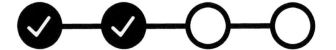

TRACKING YOUR PROGRESS

4) Taking before and after photos

This is by far the best method of accurately tracking your progress. If you look better in photo B than photo A, and all of the variables between your photos are the same, then you have 100% made progress.

I would also strongly recommend taking photos of yourself is because of how they will make you feel. Noticing the scale weight change is one thing, but seeing the changes though photos is something completely different. If you look a lot better in your second set of photos then you will honestly feel so proud of yourself!

In terms of how to take them, I would recommend showing as much skin as possible. You will most likely feel uncomfortable doing this, but it will be worth it down the line. If you wear too many clothes, it's harder to see any differences. I would also take 3 photos of yourself from different angles: the front, the side, and the back. This is because it's possible for you not to notice any difference from one angle but notice something positive from another one. I normally get my clients to pose without tensing, with their arms hanging to the side. If you're looking to build muscle, you also have the option of taking some photos of you tensing your muscles as well. If you're just looking to drop body fat though, this isn't necessary.

In terms of how often to take them, I would recommend taking them every 2-3 months. When you retake the photos, make sure that all factors are the same. This is to improve the accuracy of your conclusions. So make sure you are wearing the same clothes, and are standing in the same pose in the same room as before. Even different lighting can make a difference!

You don't have to track your progress using all four methods. However, it would lead to more accurate assessments if you did. Regardless though, taking photos of yourself is an absolute must!

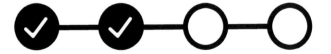

TRACKING YOUR PROGRESS

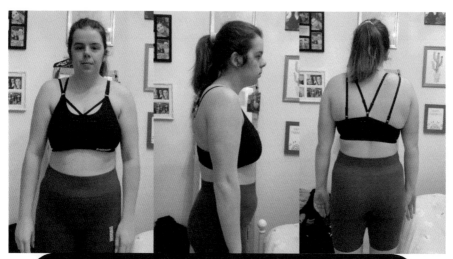

If you're a woman, I would recommend wearing a sports bra and short shorts.

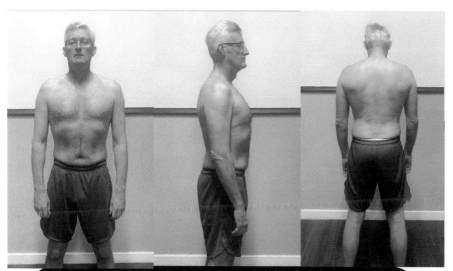

If you're a guy, I would recommend wearing just a pair of shorts.

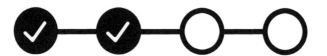

CLIENT SPOTLIGHT
GYM ANXIETY CAN BE FIXED!

ROSIE Quality Analyst Portsmouth, UK

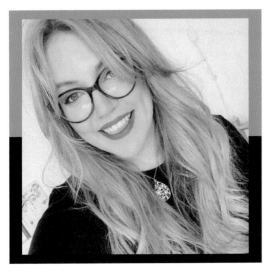

For several years, Rosie fell into bad habits and gained a lot of weight because of this. It got to the point where she was too embarrassed to even look at herself in the mirror. She knew she needed to start going to the gym, but her gym anxiety was so strong that she couldn't bring herself to do this.

One day, she managed to bite the bullet. She not only turned up, but asked for help too. In our first PT session, she was so nervous that she could barely talk to me. She hated every second of it. But I told her that if she kept coming back, things would become a lot easier for her. And they did!

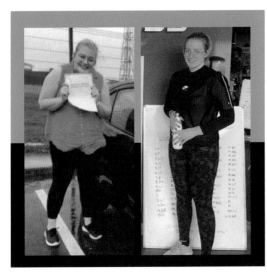

Rosie and I developed a good relationship. The comfort around me eased her nerves. She also got tremendous results from the plan that I put in place for her. She literally ended up losing 5 1/2 stone! Once she became more confident in her own body, keeping to her gym routine became an easier task.

Maybe you're reading this and you also have gym anxiety. If this is the case, know that it's a problem that can be fixed! And once it is fixed, watch your whole life change for the better.

57

CHAPTER 7:
HOW TO KNOW IF YOU'VE HAD A GOOD OR A BAD WORKOUT

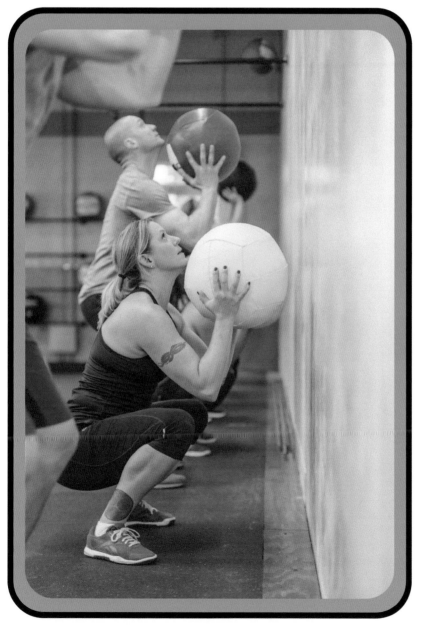

HOW TO KNOW IF YOU'VE HAD A GOOD OR A BAD WORKOUT

In a nutshell, regardless of your goal, your main priority should be improving on what you did the week before. If your goal is to gain strength, muscle or drop body fat then make sure that you're implementing progressive overload. If your goal is to improve your CV fitness, then make sure you complete your workout quicker, or perhaps increase the distance that you move. It is that simple. And again, the great thing about the gym is that you can easily quantify everything that you do. This means that it's extremely straightforward to know what you have to do in a session to move in the right direction.

However, it's just as important to talk about what's not so important. Despite not meaning too much, most people will think these are signs of a good workout:

1. Getting really hot

Surprisingly, many people think that if you get hot during a workout this is significant. In reality, it's just your body's response to stress. You can also get hot during a lot of activities, but that doesn't mean that they're good for you.

2. Getting really sweaty

Another common misconception of a good workout is getting really sweaty. The reality though, is that some people naturally sweat a lot, and others don't. Regardless, being sweaty isn't a sign of a good workout. In fact, you can have an amazing workout and not sweat very much at all. As long as you've work hard in your session and have slightly improved on the week before, then you've done your job.

HOW TO KNOW IF YOU'VE HAD A GOOD OR A BAD WORKOUT

In a nutshell, regardless of your goal, your main priority should be improving on what you did the week before. If your goal is to gain strength, muscle or drop body fat then make sure that you're implementing progressive overload. If your goal is to improve your CV fitness, then make sure you complete your workout quicker, or perhaps increase the distance that you move. It is that simple. And again, the great thing about the gym is that you can easily quantify everything that you do. This means that it's extremely straightforward to know what you have to do in a session to move in the right direction.

However, it's just as important to talk about what's not so important. Despite not meaning too much, most people will think these are signs of a good workout:

1. Getting really hot

Surprisingly, many people think that if you get hot during a workout this is significant. In reality, it's just your body's response to stress. You can also get hot during a lot of activities, but that doesn't mean that they're good for you.

2. Getting really sweaty

Another common misconception of a good workout is getting really sweaty. The reality though, is that some people naturally sweat a lot, and others don't. Regardless, being sweaty isn't a sign of a good workout. In fact, you can have an amazing workout and not sweat very much at all. As long as you've work hard in your session and have slightly improved on the week before, then you've done your job.

HOW TO KNOW IF YOU'VE HAD A GOOD OR A BAD WORKOUT

3. Burning loads of calories

Burning loads of calories in your gym workouts sounds great in theory, but the calories that you burn in the gym are only a small percentage of the total calories that you burn in a day. Therefore as I've previously mentioned, you're better off focusing on other things in your gym workouts instead.

Another reason why it's not worthwhile trying to aim to burn loads of calories is it's far easier to consume calories than to burn them. It's not worth eating 2 doughnuts if you have to run for almost an hour to try to reduce the damage done! So instead of focusing on burning calories in your sessions, try to focus on reducing the number of calories that you eat. This way you'll be more likely to lose weight, and you'll save yourself a bunch of time that you would otherwise spend on the treadmill.

4. Leaving physically destroyed

In theory, this sounds great. But if you destroy yourself so much to the point that you can't walk properly for ages, you probably went a bit overboard. If this is the case, it may take a long time for your muscles to recover. It might also mean that you have to skip an upcoming workout altogether because of this. Remember that doing 3-4 relatively high intensity workouts a week is far better than doing 1 absolutely insane one. So, if you train so hard to the point that you can't follow your program, then I would recommend reducing the intensity of your workouts a little bit.

HOW TO KNOW IF YOU'VE HAD A GOOD OR A BAD WORKOUT

5. Being really sore the day after

A lot of people enjoy being sore the day after a workout as they think it's a good sign that they've done something right. This is partially right but partially wrong. While it's definitely good to push yourself, being sore is not an indicator that you're doing anything right at all. This is because, over time, you will naturally get less and less sore even if the intensity of your workouts goes up. Therefore, you should never chase soreness. Soreness mainly occurs when you push a little bit too hard, or if you're exposed to a new stimulus. The latter scenario is why you will probably get quite sore as a beginner. This is because everything in a gym is a new stimulus! Your muscles will not be used to working this hard, meaning they will likely be sore after. After a few weeks and months though, these feelings will get less severe.

Because of what I've said here, remember that if your numbers in the gym are going up but you aren't getting sore, there is nothing to worry about!

CHAPTER 8:
KNOWING YOUR BODY

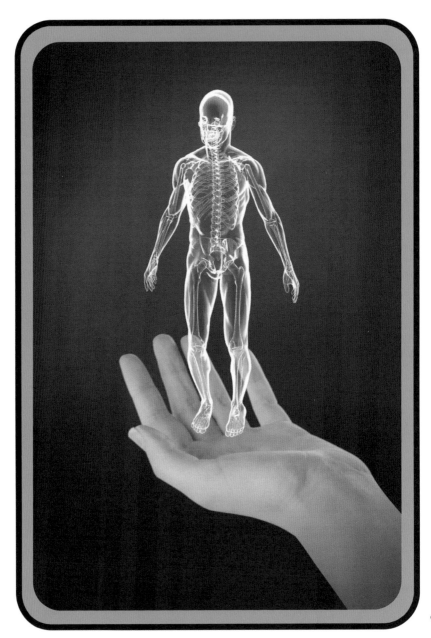

KNOWING YOUR BODY

Did you know that there are over 600 muscles in the human body? The good news though, is that you don't have to know nearly all of these. In fact, only knowing a small fraction is fine. I would try to learn all of the main muscle groups in your body, which I'm going to highlight in this section. This is important, as it's useful to know what muscles that you're meant to be working during different exercises. If you don't know this, you won't know what area that you're meant to feel pain in. A good understanding of where your muscle groups are will lead to a better chance that you'll feel exercises in the correct place.

Even though I'm only going to highlight the main muscle groups, it will still probably take you a while to learn the names of the muscles below. That's fine though. Take your time, and come back to this section when you need to. Over time, you'll naturally start to learn the names of the main muscles. Here are the muscle groups that I feel you should know. Try your best to learn them as the exercises that I'll give you in the next section involve a basic understanding of your main muscle groups.

To make things easier for you, I'm not going to refer to these areas with the longer, scientific names. Instead, I'm going to describe these areas to you with the shorter, more commonly used abbreviations.

KNOWING YOUR BODY

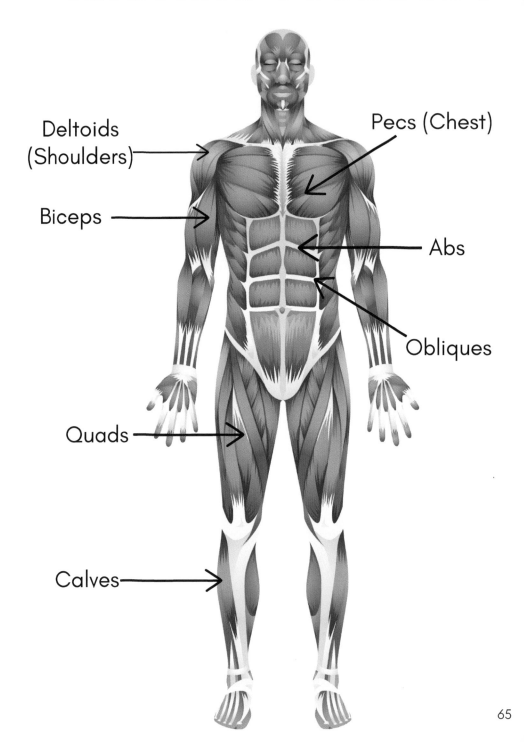

Deltoids (Shoulders)

Pecs (Chest)

Biceps

Abs

Obliques

Quads

Calves

65

KNOWING YOUR BODY

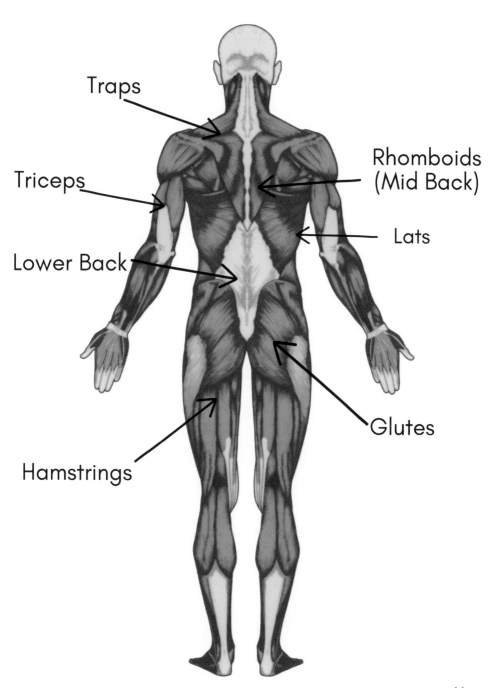

Traps

Triceps

Lower Back

Hamstrings

Rhomboids
(Mid Back)

Lats

Glutes

CLIENT SPOTLIGHT
IT'S POSSIBLE TO BREAK YOUR HABITS

ALICIA  Nurse London, UK

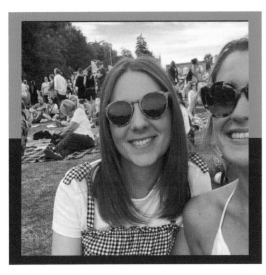

While Alicia looks after herself now, it has not always been like that.

Growing up, Alicia didn't live the healthiest of lifestyles. She ate cheap, unhealthy food. She also didn't exercise too much. Because of these things, she ended up gaining a fair bit of weight over the years.

She then decided to make a change. She started working with me and implemented all the changes that I suggested to her.

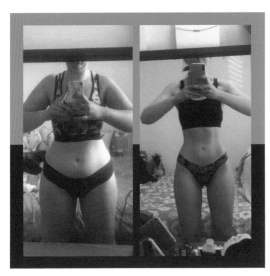

The result is that she dropped over three stone! Because she wasn't used to looking as she wanted, she suddenly felt so much happier with herself. Her confidence went up a lot, and she started to really enjoy her new lifestyle.

Just because you've let yourself go a bit, doesn't mean that you can't turn things around. Alicia is proof of this! She's in the shape of her life, and continues to improve day by day.

CHAPTER 9:
YOUR EXERCISE LIBRARY

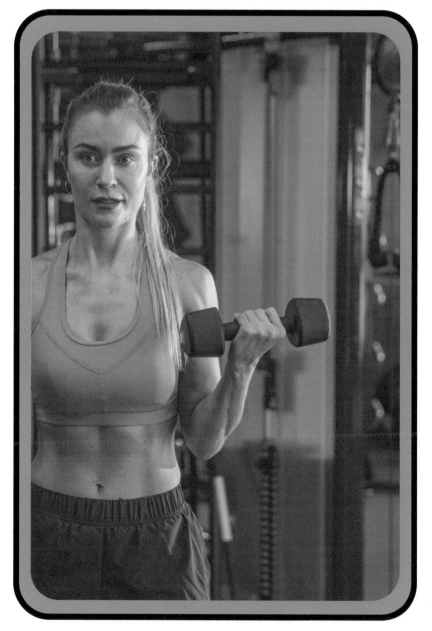

Chapter 9, Section 1: Leg Database

Section 1, Exercise 1: Plate Loaded Leg Press

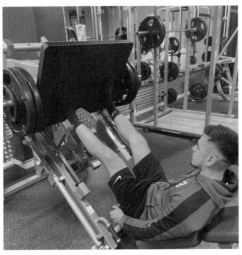

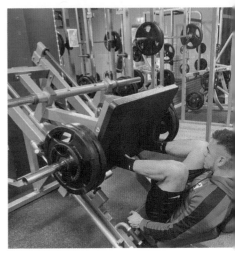

Start Position   **End Position**

Instructions:

1. Position your feet roughly shoulder width apart on the foot pad
2. Press the weight up slightly, and push the handles at the side of your hips outwards, which will unlock the machine
3. Slowly bend your knees and lower the weight down towards you, trying to achieve good depth without your hips and lower back coming up too much
4. If you're struggling to get adequate depth, try pushing your knees out away from your body on the way down, which will make room for you to go lower
5. When you're at the bottom, push the weight back up quickly until your legs are 95% straight (you can fully lock your knees instead, but if you do this make sure that you do it gently and keep the surrounding muscles tense)
6. Repeat steps 3-5

Exercise Info

Type: Compound, through the hip and knee joints
Amount of Energy Required: High
Main muscles Worked: Quads, Glutes and Hamstrings
Tempo: 3 seconds down and 1 second up

Common Mistakes:

- Make sure that your lower back doesn't come up as you lower the weight down
- Make sure that you don't do half reps, as you'll achieve better results when you go lower
- Don't forcefully lock your knees at the top, as doing so can lead to injury

Chapter 9, Section 1: Leg Database

Section 1, Exercise 2: Machine Leg Press

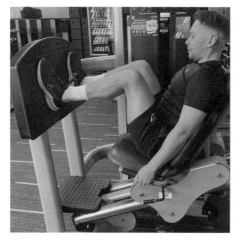

Start Position

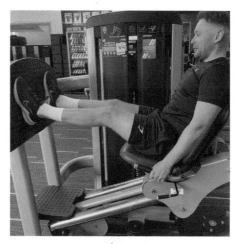

End Position

Instructions:

1. Go over to the machine and adjust the seat so it's as close to the foot pad as possible
2. Push the weight away from you quickly, this will either move the foot pad forward or the seat back depending on the make of the machine
3. Push the weight until your legs are 95% straight (you can fully lock your knees, but make sure that you do it gently and keep your surrounding muscles tense)
4. Come back in slowly
5. If you're struggling to get adequate depth, try pushing your knees out away from your body as you come back in, as this will make enough room to go a bit deeper
6. Repeat steps 2-5

Exercise Info

Type: Compound, through the hip and knee joints

Amount of Energy Required: Medium/High

Main Muscles Worked: Quads, Glutes and Hamstrings

Tempo: 1 second as you push and 3 seconds as you return the weight to the start position

Common Mistakes:

- Having the seat too far away from the foot pad when you start, it'll be too hard to achieve good depth if you do this
- Don't forcefully lock your knees at the top, as doing so could lead to injury

Chapter 9, Section 1: Leg Database
Section 1, Exercise 3: Goblet Squat

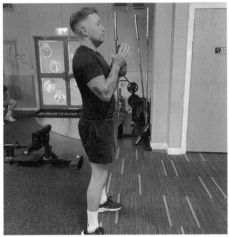

Start Position   **End Position**

Instructions:
1. Grab a kettlebell and hold it up to your chest
2. Point your toes out slightly
3. Descend slowly, making sure that you keep your chest high
4. Go down until your hips are at least in line with your knees (preferably go lower than this though if you can maintain good posture and alignment)
5. When you're at the end position, stand back up quickly until your legs are 95% straight (you can fully lock your knees at the top, but do it gently and keep your surrounding muscles tense)
6. Repeat steps 3-5

Exercise Info
Type: Compound, through the hip and knee joints
Amount of Energy Required: Medium/High
Main Muscles Worked: Quads, Glutes, Lower Back and Hamstrings
Tempo: 3 seconds down and 1 second up

Common Mistakes:
- Don't do half reps, lower the weight or take your shoes off if you are
- Don't forcefully lock your knees at the top, as doing so could lead to injury

Chapter 9, Section 1: Leg Database

Section 1, Exercise 4: Walking Dumbbell Lunges

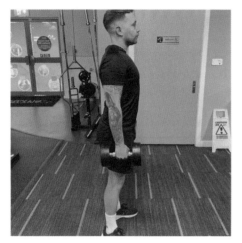 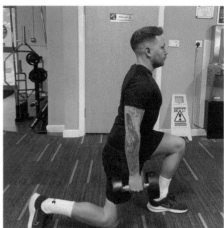

Start Position   **End Position**

Instructions:

1. Grab a set of dumbbells
2. Step forward and drop your back knee down slowly, making sure that your shoulders, hips and back knee are in a straight line as you do this
3. Keep dropping your knee down until it almost touches the floor, ending in a position where both of your legs are at right angles
4. Stand back up quickly
5. Step forward with the other foot
6. Repeat steps 2-5

Exercise Info

Type: Compound, through the hip and knee joints
Amount of Energy Required: High
Main Muscles Worked: Quads, Glutes, Lower Back and Hamstrings
Tempo: 3 seconds down and 1 second up

Common Mistakes:

- Don't forcefully lock your knees at the top, as doing so can lead to injury
- Make sure that your knee doesn't touch the floor at the bottom, as you will lose tension in your legs if this is the case
- If you get knee pain, transition to a split squat instead of this exercise (you'll find this on the next page)

Chapter 9, Section 1: Leg Database
Section 1, Exercise 5: Split Squats

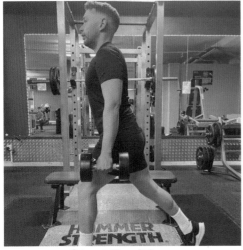

Start Position   **End Position**

Instructions:

1. Grab a set of dumbbells
2. Drop your knee down slowly, making sure that you keep your upper body relatively vertical
3. Keep dropping your knee down until it almost touches the floor, ending in a position where both of your legs are at right angles
4. Stand back up quickly
5. Repeat steps 2-4
6. Swap sides when you're done

Exercise Info

Type: Compound, through the hip and knee joints
Amount of Energy Required: Medium/High
Main Muscles Worked: Quads, Glutes, Lower Back and Hamstrings
Tempo: 3 seconds down and 1 second up

Common Mistakes:

- Don't forcefully lock your knees at the top, as doing so can lead to injury
- Make sure that your knee doesn't touch the floor at the bottom, as doing so will mean that you'll lose tension in your legs

Chapter 9, Section 1: Leg Database

Section 1, Exercise 6: Bulgarian Split Squats

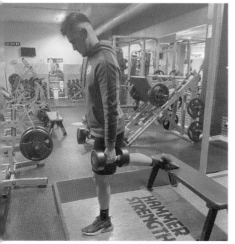
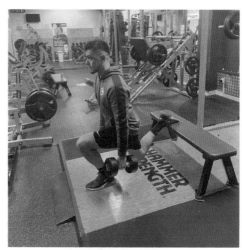

Start Position   **End Position**

Instructions:

1. Grab a set of dumbbells and go over to a bench
2. Position your toes so they're resting on the closest edge of the bench
3. Adjust your other foot so that your feet are roughly hip width apart
4. Drop your knee down and back slowly towards the bench, creating a sharp angle with this leg at the bottom
5. Go down far enough so that you feel a stretch across the front of your leg
6. From here, stand back up quickly until your leg is 95% straight (you can fully lock your knees out but do it gently and keep your surrounding muscles tense)
7. Repeat steps 4-6
8. Swap sides when you're done.

Exercise Info

Type: Compound, through the hip and knee joints

Amount of Energy Required: High

Main Muscles Worked: Quads, Glutes, Lower Back and Hamstrings

Tempo: 3 seconds down and 1 second up

Common Mistakes:

- Don't forcefully lock your knees at the top, as doing so can lead to injury
- Don't have your feet too close together
- Don't have your foot all the way back on the bench, as this will limit your ROM

Chapter 9, Section 1: Leg Database
Section 1, Exercise 7: Barbell Hip Thrusts

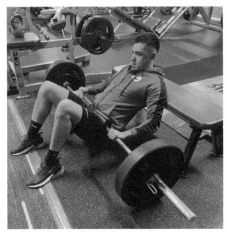

| **Start Position** | **End Position** |

Instructions:

1. Find a bench, and bring a barbell over to it. Put suitable plates on the barbell, and also place a barbell pad over the middle of it.
2. Sit on the floor in front of the bench and roll the barbell over your legs
3. When the bar is over your groin area hoist yourself up on the edge of the bench by placing your forearms on it and pushing yourself up (after this, take your arms off the bench and hold the barbell with them)
4. Slowly drop your hips down and back towards the bench, keeping your core tight and back flat
5. Thrust the weight forward and up quickly, as far as you can
6. Squeeze your glutes as hard as you can at the top
7. Repeat steps 4-6

Exercise Info

Type: Compound, hip dominant
Amount of Energy Required: High
Main Muscles Worked: Glutes and Hamstrings
Tempo: 3 seconds down and 1 second up

Common Mistakes:

- Don't have your feet too close to the bench, this will make the move feel more awkward
- Don't have too much of your back on the bench, doing so will make the move too easy

Chapter 9, Section 1: Leg Database

Section 1, Exercise 8: Romanian Deadlifts (RDL's)

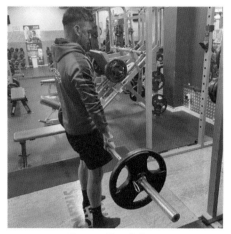
Start Position

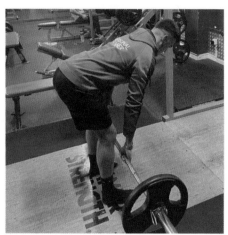
End Position

Instructions:

1. Grab a barbell and put suitable plates on it
2. While holding the bar with a shoulder width grip, initiate the move by bending over and pushing your hips back as far as you can
3. As your hips go back you want to slowly lower the bar down towards the floor (make sure the bar stays close to you the whole time that you're doing this)
4. Go down until the bar is a few inches below your knees
5. Stand up quickly to return to your starting position
6. Repeat steps 3-5

Exercise Info

Type: Compound, hip dominant
Amount of Energy Required: High
Main Muscles Worked: Glutes, Lower Back, Mid Back, Traps, Lats and Hamstrings
Tempo: 3 seconds down and 1 second up

Common Mistakes:

- Don't go too low, stop just a few inches below your knees instead
- Not pushing your hips back far enough, doing so will limit your glute activation and may result in your back rounding

Chapter 9, Section 1: Leg Database

Section 1, Exercise 9: Barbell Back Squat

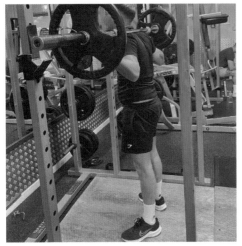

| **Start Position** | **End Position** |

Instructions:

1. Go over to a squat rack and adjust it so the bar is resting in line with your shoulders. After this, put an appropriate weight on the barbell
2. Go under the bar and rest it along your traps. Take a couple of steps back and have your feet shoulder width apart, with your toes pointing out slightly
3. Descend slowly, keeping your chest upright
4. Make sure that you go down until your hips are at least in line with your knees. Preferably go lower than this if you can though as long as you can maintain good posture
5. Stand back up quickly
6. Repeat steps 3-5

Exercise Info

Type: Compound, through the hip and knee joint

Amount of Energy Required: High

Main Muscles Worked: Quads, Glutes, Lower Back and Hamstrings

Tempo: 3 seconds down and 1 second up

Common Mistakes:

- Don't drop down really quickly, doing so can increase your risk of injury
- Letting your knees wobble throughout the move, try to keep your toes and knees in line instead

Chapter 9, Section 1: Leg Database
Section 1, Exercise 10: Smith Machine Calf Raises

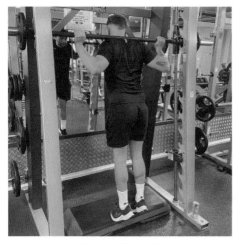

Start Position

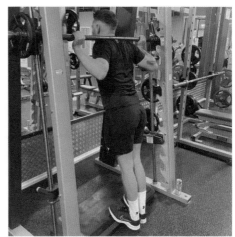

End Position

Instructions:

1. Drag some steps over to the smith machine, and place them on the floor as they're slightly in front of the bar
2. Stand with your toes on the edge of the steps
3. Go under the bar and rest it along your traps
4. Slightly raise your body up and rotate the bar forwards to unlock the machine
5. Slowly lower your body down while keeping your legs straight. Keep going down until your heels are close to the floor
6. Push yourself back up quickly and squeeze your calves at the top
7. Repeat steps 5 and 6

Exercise Info
Type: Isolation through the ankle joint
Amount of Energy Required: Low
Main Muscles Worked: Calves
Tempo: 3 seconds down and 1 second up

Common Mistakes:
- Don't do half reps with this, as that will lead to you limiting your calf activation

Chapter 9, Section 1: Leg Database

Section 1, Exercise 11: Leg Extensions

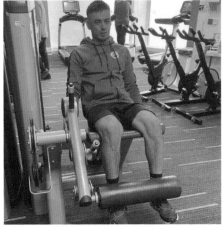
Start Position

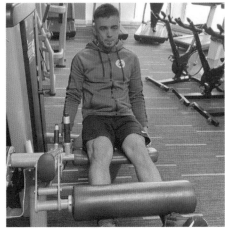
End Position

Instructions:

1. Adjust the seat so the creases of your knees are against the edge of the chair
2. Make sure that the pad is resting above your ankles
3. Keep a tall, upright body
4. Extend your legs up quickly against the weight of the pad until your shins are in line with your thighs
5. Lower the weight back down slowly to the start position
6. Repeat steps 4 and 5

Exercise Info

Type: Isolation through the knee joint
Amount of Energy Required: Medium
Main Muscles Worked: Quads
Tempo: 3 seconds down and 1 second up

Common Mistakes:

- Make sure that your hips don't come up off the chair as you extend your legs back up

Chapter 9, Section 1: Leg Database

Section 1, Exercise 12: Leg Curls

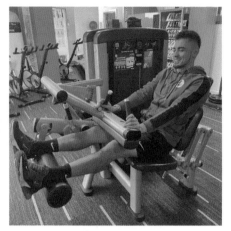

Start Position   **End Position**

Instructions:

1. Adjust the seat so one of the pads is resting just above your knees, and the other pad is resting just above your ankles
2. If that machine that you are using has handles, push into them as hard as you can to lock yourself in position
3. Drag your heels down against the weight quickly but smoothly, as far as you can
4. Raise the weight back up slowly to the start position
5. Repeat steps 3 and 4

Exercise Info	Common Mistakes:
Type: Isolation through the knee joint **Amount of Energy Required:** Medium **Main Muscles Worked:** Hamstrings **Tempo:** 1 second down and 3 seconds up	• Make sure that your hips don't come forward or that your back doesn't move off the back support (doing so will make the move easier)

Chapter 9, Section 2: Chest Database

Section 2, Exercise 1: Press Ups

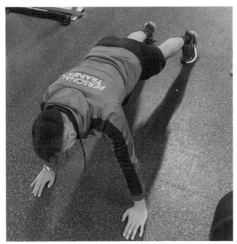
Start Position

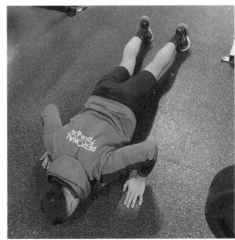
End Position

Instructions:

1. Get into a press up position, with your arms straight at the top
2. Descend your body slowly down to the floor, keeping your elbows tucked in slightly to your sides
3. Go down as far as you can, preferably going down until you get a stretch across your chest at the bottom
4. Go back up quickly all the way until your arms are straight at the top
5. Repeat steps 2-4

<table>
<tr><td>

Exercise Info

Type: Compound, through the shoulder and elbow joints
Amount of Energy Required: Medium
Main Muscles Worked: Chest, Shoulders and Triceps
Tempo: 3 seconds down and 1 second up

</td><td>

Common Mistakes:

- Flaring your elbows all the way out to the side (they should be tucked in slightly instead)
- Not going all the way down, as doing so will limit your chest activation
- Having your hips hang down lower than your chest (you should aim to keep your body in line)

</td></tr>
</table>

Chapter 9, Section 2: Chest Database
Section 2, Exercise 2: Dumbbell Chest Press

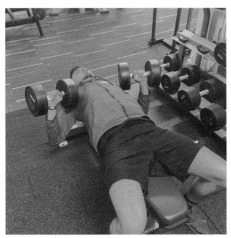

| **Start Position** | **End Position** |

Instructions:
1. Grab two dumbbells and go over to a bench
2. Set up the bench so it's flat (or at a 15-30 degree incline if you want to work your upper chest more)
3. As you descend, your elbows should be tucked into your sides slightly
4. Pull the weights down and apart slightly, make sure that you do this slowly
5. Keep going down until you feel a stretch across your chest
6. Push the dumbbells back up and in together quickly until your arms are straight
7. Repeat steps 4-6

Exercise Info
Type: Compound, through the shoulder and elbow joints
Amount of Energy Required: Medium/High
Main Muscles Worked: Chest, Shoulders and Triceps
Tempo: 3 seconds down and 1 second up

Common Mistakes:
- Flaring your elbows all the way out to the side (they should be tucked in slightly instead)
- Not going all the way down (doing so will limit your chest activation)

Chapter 9, Section 2: Chest Database
Section 2, Exercise 3: Machine Chest Press

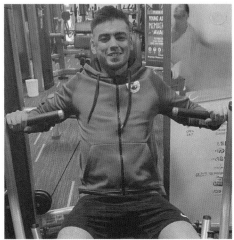

Start Position

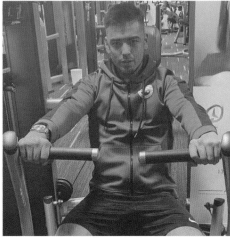

End Position

Instructions:

1. Adjust the machine so the handles that you grab are in line with your chest, and also make sure that they're set as far back as possible (so as close to your body as possible)
2. Push the handles forward quickly until you arms are straight
3. Pull them back slowly until you feel a stretch across your chest
4. Repeat steps 2 and 3

Exercise Info

Type: Compound, through the shoulder and elbow joints
Amount of Energy Required: Medium
Main Muscles Worked: Chest, Shoulders and Triceps
Tempo: 3 seconds going back and 1 second going forward

Common Mistakes:

- Not going all the way back (this will limit your chest activation)

Chapter 9, Section 2: Chest Database

Section 2, Exercise 4: Barbell Bench Press

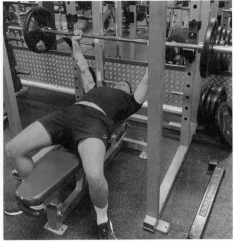

Start Position   **End Position**

Instructions:

1. Move a bench over to the middle of a rack
2. Adjust the rack so you can grab the bar and unrack it comfortably
3. Put suitable weights on the bar and lift it off the rack
4. Slowly lower the bar down until it touches your mid-chest, ideally, you should feel a stretch across your chest at the bottom
5. Push the bar up quickly until your arms are straight
6. Repeat steps 4 and 5

Exercise Info

Type: Compound, through the shoulder and elbow joints
Amount of Energy Required: Medium/High
Main Muscles Worked: Chest, Shoulders and Triceps
Tempo: 3 seconds down and 1 second up

Common Mistakes:

- Bouncing the weight off your chest, instead you need to go down slowly to fully activate your chest and avoid injury
- Not touching your chest with the bar, as this will again result in you not fully activating your chest

Chapter 9, Section 2: Chest Database

Section 2, Exercise 5: Machine Chest Fly

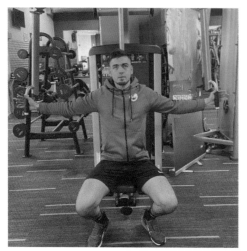

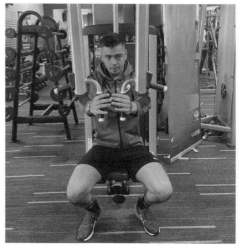

Start Position　　　　　　　　**End Position**

Instructions:

1. Adjust the machine so your chest is in line with the handles
2. Bring the weights in together quickly with a slight bend in your arms
3. Bring the weights slowly back until you feel a stretch across your chest at the back
4. When you feel that stretch, bring the weight back in together quickly
5. Repeat steps 2-4

Exercise Info

Type: Isolation through the shoulder joint
Amount of Energy Required: Medium/Low
Main Muscles Worked: Chest
Tempo: 3 seconds as you bring the weight back and 1 second as you bring the weight forward

Common Mistakes:

- Not feeling the stretch across your chest at the back (if this is the case then you won't activate your chest as much as you could)
- Having your arms too bent, doing so will make the move easier

Chapter 9, Section 3: Back Database
Section 3, Exercise 1: Assisted Pull Ups

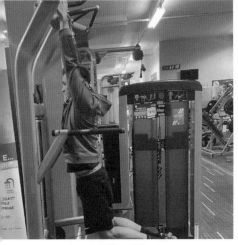

Start Position

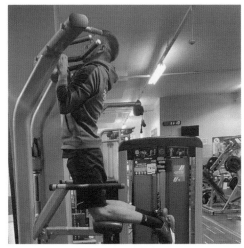

End Position

Instructions:

1. Go over to the assisted pull up machine
2. Put your knees up so they are on the pad
3. There are plenty of different ways to grab the bars at the top, but I would recommend a narrow grip for the time being (this is typically how most people do best)
4. Pull your body up quickly but smoothly until your chin is in line with the handles at the top (lean back very slightly with your upper back as you do this)
5. Slowly lower yourself back down to the starting position until your arms are straight, and bring your upper body forward slightly as you approach the bottom
6. Repeat steps 4 and 5

Exercise Info

Type: Compound, through the shoulder and elbow joints
Amount of Energy Required: Medium/High
Main Muscles Worked: Mid Back, Traps, Lats, Shoulders and Biceps
Tempo: 3 seconds down and 1 second up

Common Mistakes:

- Not fully straightening your arms at the bottom (doing this will mean you don't get a stretch in your lats, meaning your back isn't doing the amount of work that it could be doing)
- Not remembering the weights are reversed with this machine (the lighter the weight on here, the harder it is)

Chapter 9, Section 3: Back Database

Section 3, Exercise 2: Cable Row

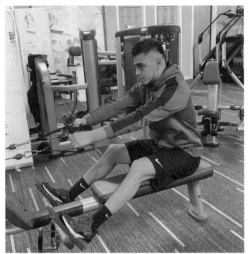

Start Position

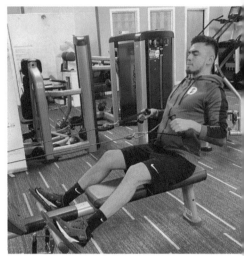

End Position

Instructions:

1. Go over to the cable row machine
2. Place your feet on the foot rest and keep your knees slightly bent
3. Grab the handle and drag it towards your stomach quickly, leaning back slightly with your upper back as you do this.
4. Keep bringing your arms back until your elbows are slightly past your body
5. Straighten your arms slowly, leaning forward with your upper back as you do this
6. Repeat steps 3-5

Exercise Info

Type: Isolation through the shoulder joint
Amount of Energy Required: Medium/High
Main Muscles Worked: Mid Back, Traps, Lats, Shoulders and Biceps
Tempo: 3 seconds as you bring the weight forward and 1 second as you bring the weight back

Common Mistakes:

- Keeping your back stationary the whole time (if you don't move your back slightly with your arms, then you'll limit your back activation)
- Moving your back too much (if this is the case, then the move will become too easy)

Chapter 9, Section 3: Back Database
Section 3, Exercise 3: Lat Pull Down

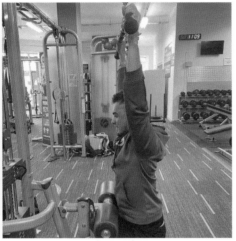

| **Start Position** | **End Position** |

Instructions:

1. Go over to the lat pulldown machine and adjust the pads so you can trap your thighs underneath them
2. There are a few ways you can hold the bar, but typically just grab it with a shoulder width grip and with your palms facing forwards
3. Drag the weight down quickly but smoothly to your upper chest level (as you do this, lean back slightly with your upper back)
4. After the bar touches your upper chest, straighten your arms back over you slowly (as you do this, lean forward slightly with your upper body)
5. Repeat steps 3 and 4

Exercise Info
Type: Compound, through the shoulder and elbow joints
Amount of Energy Required: Medium
Main Muscles Worked: Mid Back, Traps, Lats, Shoulders and Biceps
Tempo: 3 seconds up and 1 second down

Common Mistakes:
- Not straightening your arms at the top (if this is the case then you won't get a stretch in your lats, leading to the exercise becoming too easy)
- Bringing the weight down so it's too far in front of you (if you do this, you'll start to change the target muscles)

Chapter 9, Section 3: Back Database
Section 3, Exercise 4: One Arm Dumbbell Row

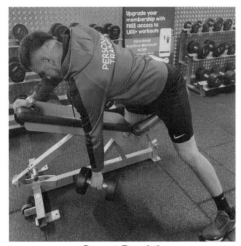

Start Position

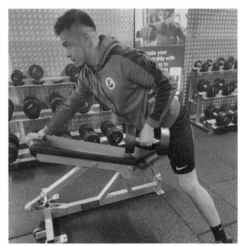

End Position

Instructions:

1. Grab one dumbbell and head over to a bench
2. Adjust the bench so it's between 0 and 30 degrees
3. Put one knee in the gap in the bench, and the same hand at the top of the bench
4. Put your opposite leg straight out to the side, and grab the dumbbell with the same hand
5. Push your hips back and lift your chest up
6. Drag the dumbbell up quickly but smoothly until your elbow is slightly past your body
7. Slowly lower the weight down, leaning that half of your body down to the floor as the dumbbell travels down
8. Repeat steps 6 and 7
9. Swap sides

Exercise Info

Type: Compound, through the shoulder and elbow joints
Amount of Energy Required: Medium/High
Main Muscles Worked: Mid Back, Traps, Lats, Shoulders and Biceps
Tempo: 3 seconds down and 1 second up

Common Mistakes:

- Shrugging your shoulder up as you drag the dumbbell up (doing so will engage your traps too much, limiting the work that the rest of your back has to do)
- Not leaning down with your upper body as you lower the dumbbell (doing so will result in your back not activating as much as it could)

Chapter 9, Section 3: Back Database
Section 3, Exercise 5: Standing One Arm Cable Row

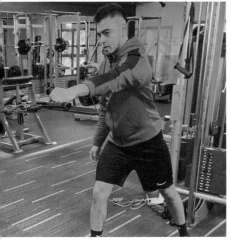

Start Position

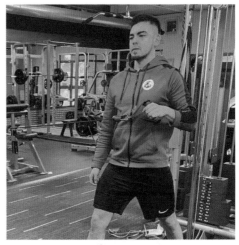

End Position

Instructions:
1. Go over to the cable machine and attach a handle to it
2. Move the cable up so it's roughly in line with your chest
3. Grab the handle with one arm and move your opposite foot forward, keeping the other foot back
4. Drag your elbow back quickly until it's past your body (as you do this lean back with your upper back slightly)
5. Straight your arm slowly and slightly lean forward with that side of your body
6. Repeat steps 4 and 5
7. Swap sides

Exercise Info
Type: Compound, through the shoulder and elbow joints
Amount of Energy Required: Medium
Main Muscles Worked: Mid Back, Traps, Lats, Shoulders and Biceps
Tempo: 3 seconds as you bring the weight forward and 1 second as you bring the weight back

Common Mistakes:
- Shrugging your shoulder too far back as you move your arm back (doing so will result in your traps doing too much work)
- Not staggering your feet (doing so will mean you'll struggle for balance)

Chapter 9, Section 4: Shoulder Database
Section 4, Exercise 1: Standing Barbell Shoulder Press

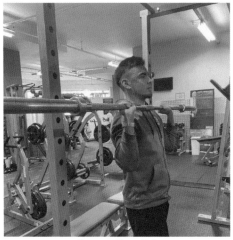

Start Position

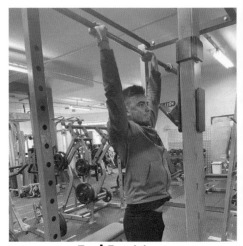

End Position

Instructions:

1. Go over to a rack and set the bar up so it's in line with your upper chest
2. Grab the bar with a shoulder width grip, with your palms facing away from you
3. Step back with the bar in your hands, resting it around your collarbone
4. Stagger your stance for balance
5. Press the weight quickly up over your head until your arms are straight (as you do this, push your head through and the bar behind you slightly)
6. Lower the bar slowly until it's at your upper chest level again
7. Repeat steps 5 and 6

Exercise Info

Type: Compound, through the shoulder and elbow joints
Amount of Energy Required: Medium/High
Main Muscles Worked: Shoulders, Triceps and Traps
Tempo: 3 seconds down and 1 second up

Common Mistakes:

- Pressing the weight too far in front of you (you'll be stronger when you keep it over the middle of your head, so press the bar back slightly as you press it into the air)
- Not tensing your core throughout (if this is the case, you may arch your back too much)

Chapter 9, Section 4: Shoulder Database
Section 4, Exercise 2: Machine Shoulder Press

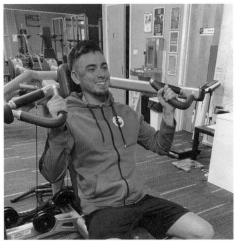

Start Position

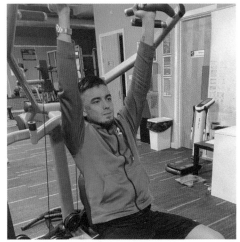

End Position

Instructions:
1. Go over to the shoulder press machine and adjust the machine so the handles start just above your shoulder height
2. Press the handles up quickly until your arms are straight at the top
3. Slowly lower the handles back down until you reach your shoulder height
4. Repeat steps 2 and 3

Exercise Info
Type: Compound, through the shoulder and elbow joints
Amount of Energy Required: Medium
Main Muscles Worked: Shoulders, Triceps and Traps
Tempo: 3 seconds down and 1 second up

Common Mistakes:
- Don't bring the handles all the way down (if the weights touch again, then you'll lose tension so only go about 95% down instead)

Chapter 9, Section 4: Shoulder Database
Section 4, Exercise 3: Seated Dumbbell Shoulder Press

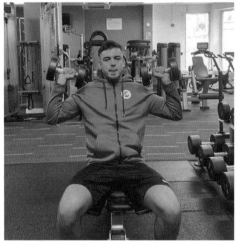

Start Position

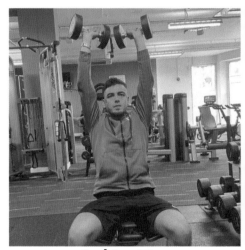

End Position

Instructions:

1. Grab a pair of dumbbells and go over to a bench
2. Set the bench up so it's around 75 degrees
3. After sitting on the bench, press the dumbbells up and in together quickly until your arms are straight (try to keep the weights over the middle of your head as you do this)
4. After that, slowly lower them back down until they're just above your shoulder level
5. Repeat steps 3 and 4

Exercise Info

Type: Compound, through the shoulder and elbow joints
Amount of Energy Required: Medium/High
Main Muscles Worked: Shoulders, Triceps and Traps
Tempo: 3 seconds down and 1 second up

Common Mistakes:

- Arching your back too much as you lift the weight up (try to suck your belly button into your stomach as you lift the weight up)
- Pressing the weights too far in front of you, as you'll be weaker if you do this

Chapter 9, Section 4: Shoulder Database
Section 4, Exercise 4: Assisted Dips

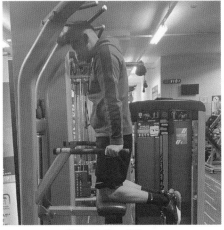

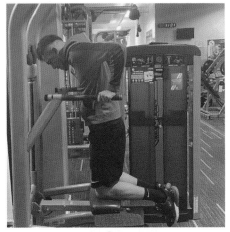

Start Position   **End Position**

Instructions:

1. Go over to the assisted dip machine
2. Grip the handlebars, making sure that they're roughly shoulder width apart
3. Bring your knees up on the pad
4. Slowly lower your body down until your shoulders are in line with your elbows
5. Press yourself up quickly until your arms are straight at the top
6. Repeat steps 4 and 5

Exercise Info	Common Mistakes:
Type: Compound, through the shoulder and elbow joints **Amount of Energy Required:** Medium/High **Main Muscles Worked:** Shoulders, Triceps, Chest and Traps **Tempo:** 3 seconds down and 1 second up	• Not going low enough, (this will result in the move being too easy) • Not remembering the weights are reversed on this machine (the lighter the weight, the easier it is)

Chapter 9, Section 4: Shoulder Database
Section 4, Exercise 5: Machine Rear Delt Fly

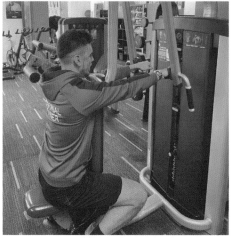

Start Position

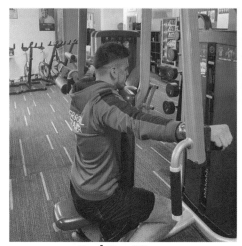

End Position

Instructions:

1. Go over to the rear delt fly machine and adjust it so the handles are in line with your shoulders
2. Keep your arms slightly bent
3. Keeping your chest against the pad, bring the handles out quickly to the side until they're around 3/4 of the way back
4. Slowly bring the handles back to the starting position
5. Repeat steps 3 and 4

Exercise Info

Type: Isolation through the shoulder joint
Amount of Energy Required: Low
Main Muscles Worked: Shoulders and Traps
Tempo: 3 seconds as you bring the weight forward and 1 second as you bring the weight back

Common Mistakes:

- Going too far back (with this exercise, other parts of your body will take over if this is the case)

Chapter 9, Section 4: Shoulder Database
Section 4, Exercise 6: Cable Face Pull

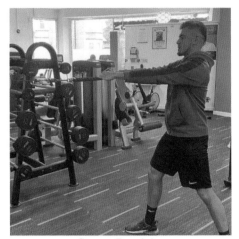 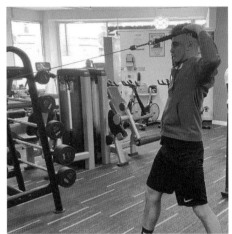

Start Position   **End Position**

Instructions:

1. Go over to the cable and attach a rope to it
2. Move the cable up so the rope is in line with your upper chest level
3. Grab each end of the rope with your palms facing each other
4. Take a few steps away from the cable machine, then stagger your stance
5. Pull the rope quickly in towards your forehead, as far as you can
6. As you do this bring your elbows back and keep them in line with your shoulders (you want to end in a double bicep flex pose)
7. Bring the weight slowly back in towards the cable
8. Repeat steps 5-7

Exercise Info

Type: Isolation through the shoulder joint
Amount of Energy Required: Low
Main Muscles Worked: Shoulders and Traps
Tempo: 3 seconds as you bring the weight forward and 1 second as you bring the weight back

Common Mistakes:

- Having your feet in line with each other (you'll be more balanced if you stagger your stance instead)

Chapter 9, Section 4: Shoulder Database
Section 4, Exercise 7: Dumbbell Side Lateral Raises

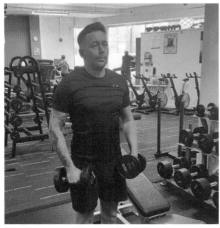 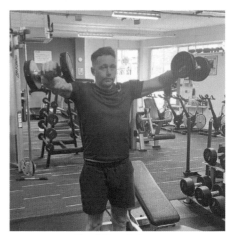

Start Position   **End Position**

Instructions:

1. Grab two dumbbells
2. Lift them up in a diagonal line quickly, trying to aim your hands towards the corners of the room that you're in (keep a slight bend in your arms as you do this)
3. Keep going up until your hands are in line with your shoulders
4. Slowly lower the weights back down to the starting position
5. Repeat steps 3 and 4

Exercise Info
Type: Isolation through the shoulder joint
Amount of Energy Required: Low
Main Muscles Worked: Shoulders and Traps
Tempo: 3 seconds down and 1 second up

Common Mistakes:
- Moving your back throughout the move (if you do this then you'll use momentum to help get the weight up, limiting the work that your shoulders have to do)

Chapter 9, Section 5: Arm Database
Section 5, Exercise 1: Incline Dumbbell Curls

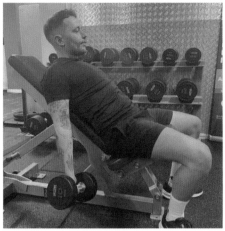

| **Start Position** | **End Position** |

Instructions:
1. Grab two dumbbells and go over to a bench
2. Set the bench up so it's between 45 and 60 degrees
3. Lie down on the bench with your arms hanging to your side (make sure that your elbows are behind your body)
4. Your hands should be holding the pair of dumbbells, with your palms facing forwards
5. Curl the dumbbells quickly up to your upper chest level, keeping your elbows still
6. Keeping your elbows still again, lower the weight down slowly until your arms are straight
7. Repeat steps 5 and 6

Exercise Info
Type: Isolation through the elbow joint
Amount of Energy Required: Low
Main Muscles Worked: Biceps
Tempo: 3 seconds down and 1 second up

Common Mistakes!
- Not straightening your arms at the bottom (doing this will limit the work that your biceps have to do)
- Swinging your elbows throughout the move (doing so will mean that you use momentum to get the weight up, rather than your strength)

Chapter 9, Section 5: Arm Database
Section 5, Exercise 2: Standing Dumbbell Hammer Curls

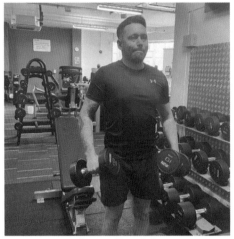

Start Position	End Position

Instructions:

1. Grab two dumbbells
2. Make sure that your palms are facing each other as you hold the dumbbells
3. Curl the dumbbells up and in together quickly, up to your upper chest level (make sure that your elbows are still as you do this and keep your palms facing inwards)
4. Bring the dumbbells back down slowly until your arms are straight, making sure that your elbows are in the same position
5. Repeat steps 3 and 4

Exercise Info

Type: Isolation through the elbow joint
Amount of Energy Required: Low
Main Muscles Worked: Biceps
Tempo: 3 seconds down and 1 second up

Common Mistakes:

- Not straightening your arms at the bottom (doing this will limit the work that your biceps have to do)
- Moving your back as well as your arms (if you back swing, you'll use momentum to get the weight up instead of your strength)

Chapter 9, Section 5: Arm Database
Section 5, Exercise 3: Cable Straight Bar Curls

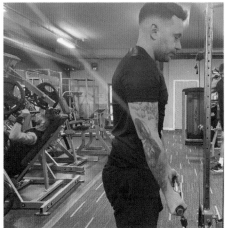

Start Position

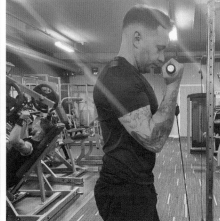

End Position

Instructions:

1. Go over to a cable machine
2. Put the cable all the way to the bottom, and attach a straight bar to it
3. Curl the weight up quickly to your upper chest height, keeping your elbows still the whole time
4. Straighten your arms back down slowly
5. Repeat steps 3 and 4

Exercise Info
Type: Isolation through the elbow joint
Amount of Energy Required: Low
Main Muscles Worked: Biceps
Tempo: 3 seconds down and 1 second up

Common Mistakes!
- Not straightening your arms at the bottom (doing this will limit the work that your biceps have to do)
- Moving your back as well as your arm (if you back swing, you'll use momentum to get the weight up instead of your strength)

Chapter 9, Section 5: Arm Database
Section 5, Exercise 4: Dumbbell Skull Crushers

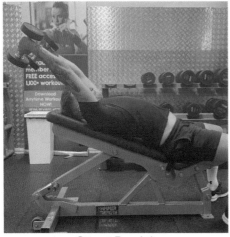
Start Position

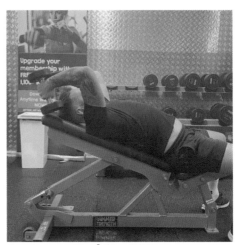
End Position

Instructions:
1. Grab a set of dumbbells and go over to a bench and set it up so it's between 0 and 30 degrees
2. Lie with your back on the bench, with your head at the top of it
3. Extend your arms up into the air above you until your arms are straight (after this, shift your elbows back slightly)
4. Dip the dumbbells slowly down towards your head
5. Go down far enough so you feel a stretch in your triceps
6. When you're at that point, extend back up quickly until your arms are straight
7. Repeat steps 4-6

Exercise Info
Type: Isolation through the elbow joint
Amount of Energy Required: Low
Main Muscles Worked: Triceps
Tempo: 3 seconds down and 1 second up

Common Mistakes:
- Not having your elbows back enough (if they're too far forwards, you won't work your triceps as much as you could)

Chapter 9, Section 5: Arm Database
Section 5, Exercise 5: Overhead Rope Cable Extensions

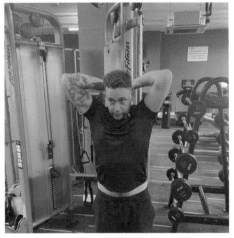

| **Start Position** | **End Position** |

Instructions:

1. Go over to a cable machine
2. Put the cable all the way to the bottom, and attach a rope to it
3. Grab the rope with your palms facing each other, and twist to face away from the cable
4. Bring the weight up to your head level with your elbows as far behind you as possible
5. From here, extend the rope up and apart quickly until your arms are straight (keep your elbows still as you do this)
6. Keeping your elbows still again, slowly lower the weight down until the rope is behind your head (go down far enough so you feel a stretch in your triceps)
7. Repeat steps 5 and 6

Exercise Info

Type: Isolation through the elbow joint
Amount of Energy Required: Low
Main Muscles Worked: Triceps
Tempo: 3 seconds down and 1 second up

Common Mistakes:

- Having your elbows too far forwards (you need them as far back/up into the air as possible)

Chapter 9, Section 5: Arm Database
Section 5, Exercise 6: Tricep Pushdowns

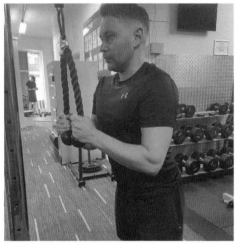

| **Start Position** | **End Position** |

Instructions:

1. Go over to a cable machine
2. Put the cable all the way to the top, and attach a rope
3. Grab the rope with your palms facing each other, and slightly lean forward with your upper body
4. From here, extend the rope down and apart quickly until your arms are straight (keep your elbows still as you do this, and get your hands to the side of your legs)
5. Keeping your elbows still again, slowly raise the weight back up to the start position
6. Repeat steps 4 and 5

Exercise Info
Type: Isolation through the elbow joint
Amount of Energy Required: Low
Main Muscles Worked: Triceps
Tempo: 3 seconds up and 1 second down

Common Mistakes:
- Moving your elbows forward as you raise the weight back up, your forearms should be the only part of you moving
- Not fully straightening your arms at the bottom (this will make the move too easy)

Chapter 9, Section 6: Core Database
Section 6, Exercise 1: V Ups

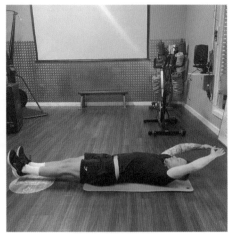 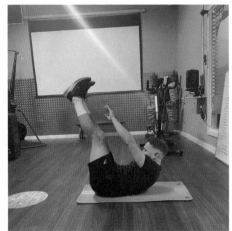

Start Position   **End Position**

Instructions:

1. Go over to a mat
2. Lie on your back on the mat
3. Raise your legs and arms up together quickly until they meet above your core, in the middle of your body
4. Slowly lower them both back down to the starting position, trying to keep your legs from touching the floor again at the bottom
5. Repeat steps 3 and 4

Exercise Info

Type: Isolation through the hip joint
Amount of Energy Required: Low
Main Muscles Worked: Abs
Tempo: 3 seconds down and 1 second up

Common Mistakes:

- Touching the floor with your feet at the bottom of each rep (if you do this, you'll lose the tension that you've built up in your core)

Chapter 9, Section 6: Core Database
Section 6, Exercise 2: Plank

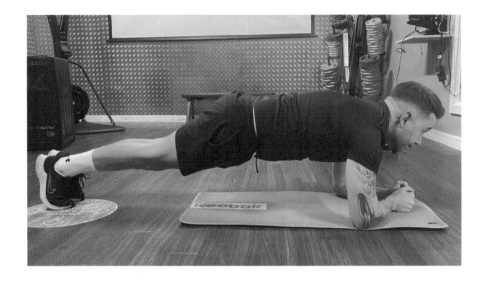

Instructions:

1. Go over to a mat
2. Face the floor and place your elbows directly below your shoulders
3. Raise your body up so that you're resting just on your toes and your forearms, keeping your body in a reasonably straight line
4. Round your upper back slightly
5. Try to suck your belly button into your stomach
6. Squeeze your glutes
7. Hold yourself in that position for as long as you can

Exercise Info

Type: Isolation, static hold
Amount of Energy Required: Low
Main Muscles Worked: Deeper core muscles

Common Mistakes:

- Having your hips too low or too high, either option will result in less core activation
- Arching your lower back (try to suck your belly button in towards your spine to help with this)

Chapter 9, Section 6: Core Database
Section 6, Exercise 3: Cable Woodchoppers

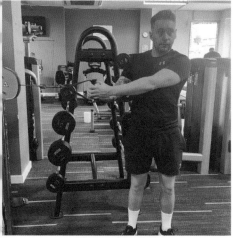

Start Position

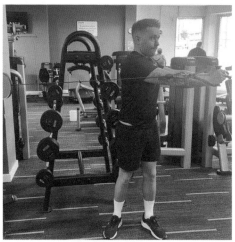

End Position

Instructions:

1. Go over to the cable machine
2. Attach a handle to it, and adjust the machine so the cable is around your lower chest level
3. Stand side on to the cable and grab the handle, then shuffle sideways away from the cable, for a few steps
4. Press the weight out on in front of you with your arms straight
5. Twist your body and the weight away from the machine quickly
6. Slowly twist your body and the weight back towards the cable
7. Repeat steps 5 and 6
8. Swap sides

Exercise Info
Type: Isolation through the hip joint
Amount of Energy Required: Low
Main Muscles Worked: Obliques and deeper core muscles
Tempo: 1 second as you twist away from the cable and 3 seconds as you twist back towards it

Common Mistakes:
- Bending your arms too much (keep the weight far from you at all times instead)
- Standing too close to the cable (when you twist the weight back towards the cable, the weight should not fully reset)

106

Chapter 9, Section 7: Cardio Database
Section 7, Exercise 1: Treadmill

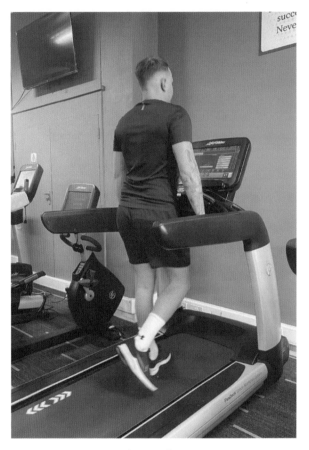

Instructions:

1. Go over to a treadmill
2. Press one of the green 'Go' or 'Start' buttons
3. Identify the emergency stop feature of the treadmill, just in case you have to use it if you're struggling to keep the right pace later on in your workout
4. To change the speed of the treadmill, you should look for a running man with a '+' and a '-' around it
5. To change the incline of the treadmill, look for a picture of a man running up a hill with a '+' and a '-' sign around it (the higher the incline, the harder it will be)
6. Check out the screen to see how many calories you've burnt, the speed at which you're running and more features
7. To stop, press the red 'stop button'

Chapter 9, Section 7: Cardio Database
Section 7, Exercise 2: Cross Trainer

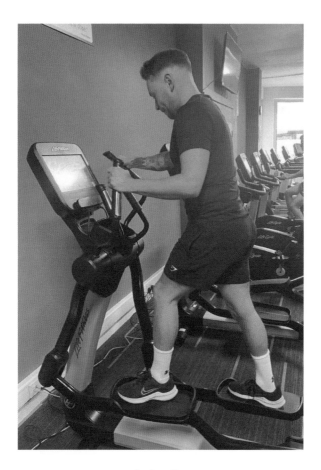

Instructions:

1. Go over to the cross trainer
2. Press one of the green 'Go' or 'Start' buttons
3. Hold onto the handles and keep your chest up
4. You want to actively use your upper body to push and pull the handlebars to and from your body
5. As you do this, move your legs forward and down in a circular type motion
6. To change the speed of the cross trainer, look for a running man with a '+' and a '-' around it
7. To change the incline of the cross trainer, look for a picture of a man running up a hill with a '+' and a '-' sign around it (the higher the incline, the harder it will be)
8. Check out the screen to see how many calories you've burnt, the speed at which you're running and more features
9. To stop, press the red 'stop button'

Chapter 9, Section 7: Cardio Database
Section 7, Exercise 3: Bicycle

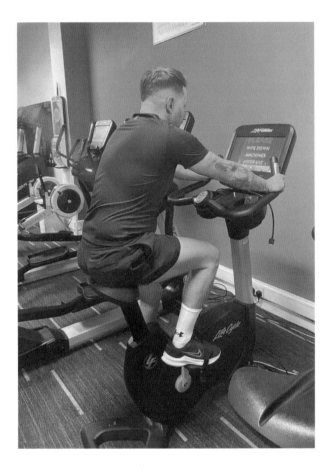

Instructions:

1. Go over to the bicycle
2. Adjust the seat height so its roughly in line with your hips
3. Safely get onto the bicycle by putting one foot in one of the pedals, one hand on one of the handles, and the other hand on the seat to help you climb up
4. Start pedalling (some bicycle machines will start automatically when you do this but if yours doesn't, then press one of the green 'Go' or 'Start' buttons)
5. Check to see if the seat is in the right place (if you can fully straighten your legs at the bottom, then the seat needs to be moved down slightly)
6. To change the speed of the bicycle, look for a running man with a '+' and a '-' around it
7. To change the incline of the bicycle, look for a picture of a man running up a hill with a '+' and a '-' sign around it (the higher the incline, the harder it will be)
8. Check out the screen to see how many calories you've burnt, the speed at which you're cycling and more features
9. To stop, press the red 'stop button'

Chapter 9, Section 7: Cardio Database
Section 7, Exercise 4: Rowing Machine

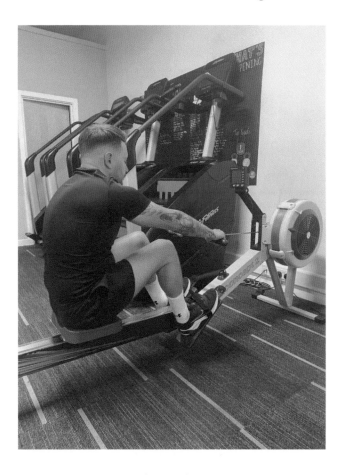

Instructions:

1. Go over to the rowing machine
2. Select the resistance that you'd like to use (this should be a feature of the machine where there is a scale between 1 and 10, with an arrow that you can move to pick the number)
3. Set up the foot straps to cross comfortably over the front of your foot
4. Turn the machine on by either pressing the 'go' button, or the menu button (if it's the latter option, click 'just row' afterwards)
5. Grab the handle
6. Push away from the machine with your legs and as you do this, pull the handle towards your ribs
7. As your legs are almost straight, lean back slightly with your upper body
8. After this, straighten your arms and bring the handle back towards the machine (as you do this bring your hips forward and bend your knees, trying to bring the seat as far forward as you can)
9. To stop, put the handle back where it was prior to engaging in this exercise

Chapter 9, Section 8: Stretching Database

For the sole purpose of not making this book being too long, I won't go into detail outlining all of the different types of stretches that you can do. This is just because there are so many different stretches to potentially cover. If one of your one main goals is to improve your mobility, feel free to contact me and I'll offer you some suggestions on what to do. You will find my contact details at the end of this book.

CLIENT SPOTLIGHT
DON'T LET YOUR METABOLISM HOLD YOU BACK!

ELLIOTT Teacher Singapore

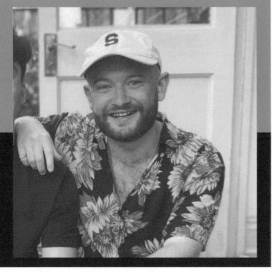

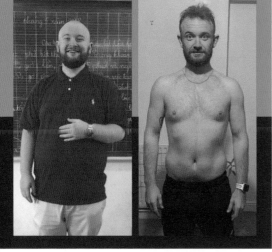

Elliott has been one of my closest friends for the last decade. During this time, he's struggled a lot with his weight. He was born with a naturally slow metabolism and found it very easy to gain body fat if he made bad choices.

I wanted to change this, so asked if he would be interested in working with me. He agreed, and I put a plan in place for him.

The result was that he trimmed down, and built up some muscle too. Because of this, his confidence increased dramatically. His motivation and desire to keep the process going also strengthened, as he knew the plan was working.

For those of you who have a slow metabolism, there is absolutely no doubt that you have it harder than most people! But that doesn't mean that you're doomed. You just need a good plan in place and you need to be more consistent than the average person. If this is the case, you'll be just fine.

CHAPTER 11:
HOW TO STRUCTURE YOUR WEEK

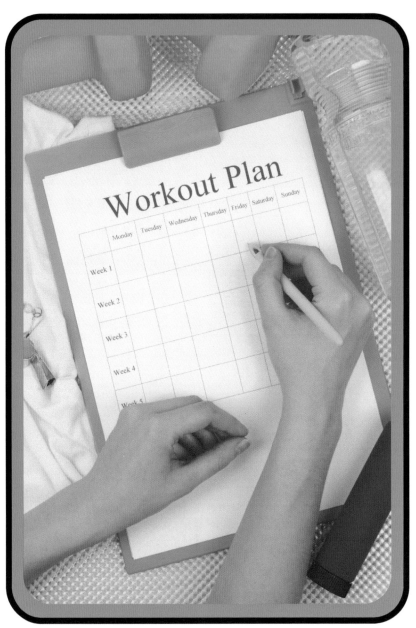

How To Structure Your Week

Just like how there is no perfect "one size fits all" workout, there is no perfect way to structure your week either. The main factor that determines your workout split is deciding how many days you want to commit to going to the gym each week. If you commit to going 5 or 6 days a week, you have the option of splitting up your muscle groups more across the week. On the other hand, if you only go 2 or 3 days a week, then you will not have the time available to do this.

What you need to do is make sure that you hit each of your main muscle groups between 2 and 4 times a week. This specific number will depend on how big the muscle is. If they're small muscles, like the back of your shoulders (rear deltoids), you can hit them up to 4 times a week. If it's a bigger muscle, like the front of your thighs (quadriceps) then 2 to 3 times is more suitable. Regardless, if you want good results, then every single muscle must be worked a minimum of twice a week.

People who don't do this are destined for slow progress. In fact, how to structure your week is one of the most important variables that will decide your success. Splits that lead to you only hitting each of your muscles once a week are commonly referred to as 'bro splits'. Here is an example of one:

Monday: Chest
Tuesday: Back
Wednesday: Shoulders
Thursday: Arms
Friday: Legs
Saturday: Rest
Sunday: Rest

How To Structure Your Week

Beginners are particularly prone to following a workout split like this. This is because they don't yet have a good understanding of how to train. And like I said earlier, you will progress the quickest when you hit all of your muscles between 2 and 4 times a week. So, imagine if you do genuinely still want to train one muscle a session. Here is what your week would have to look like to accomplish that:

Monday morning: Chest
Monday afternoon: Legs
Tuesday morning: Back
Tuesday afternoon: Arms
Wednesday morning: Shoulders
Wednesday afternoon: Calves
Thursday morning: Arms
Thursday afternoon: Chest
Friday morning: Legs
Friday afternoon: Shoulders
Saturday: Calves
Sunday: Rest

As you can see, to achieve the recommended frequency, you would in theory need to workout twice a day almost every single day of the week. Do you want to do that? Do you even have the time to do that? So please make sure that you don't follow this common error. Unless you want to live in the gym, never go into the gym just to hit one muscle at a time!

How To Structure Your Week

Now I've told you what to do and what not to do, here's why I'm saying these things. Earlier in this book, I told you that if your goal is to either build muscle or lose weight, weight training is the best form of training for you, as it will force your muscles to change. One of the best ways to do that is not only by working them hard, but also by hitting them frequently. This is because muscles change through a process called muscle protein synthesis. This is basically the muscle-building process. The problem is, muscle protein synthesis only occurs in the 48 hours after you train that particular muscle. For instance, let's say that you only train chest once a week on Mondays. After Wednesday, that muscle isn't changing anymore. So, you literally waste the next 5 days of the week! Whereas, if you train your chest twice a week, that muscle is changing 4 days of the week instead of 2. Hopefully, this example makes you realize that only hitting each muscle once a week is a big problem. So, make sure you don't do this! A higher frequency approach will always lead to better results.

Another benefit to a higher frequency approach is that you can afford to be in the gym less often. Lots of us lead busy lives, and we realistically don't want to be in the gym all the time. If you do use a high frequency split though, it means that you can afford to only go to the gym between 2 and 4 times a week. This is the approach that I tend to use with most of my clients. If I tell them that they only have to be in the gym for that amount of time, they're more likely to do all of their sessions. It also means that they can live a fun lifestyle alongside their training.

Now, let's dive into some great workout splits! I'm going to highlight some different splits below. First, decide how many days you are willing to commit to the gym a week, and then look at my tailored advice for you!

How To Structure Your Week

1. 2 days a week

If you only want to work out twice a week, then you should be doing full body sessions. This way, you can still hit all your main muscles twice a week, meaning that you still fall into that ideal frequency range. Even though 2 days a week in the gym isn't a lot, you can surprisingly still make some decent progress, while maximizing the lifestyle you can live outside of it. If this sounds good to you, I would recommend that you leave 3 days between the 2 workouts.

Here's what your routine might look like:
Monday: Full Body
Tuesday: Rest
Wednesday: Rest
Thursday: Full Body
Friday: Rest
Saturday: Rest
Sunday: Rest

P R O S

- Extremely time efficient
- You still fall into the optimal frequency range if you do full body sessions
- You have your weekends free for social activities
- Because you don't go to the gym that often, you will never be affected
- by fatigue issues

C O N S

- Not much time to incorporate any isolation movements, meaning you may develop lagging muscle groups
- It's a minimalist approach: you will not develop your muscles groups as quickly as you would if you went to the gym more days a week
- Because leg training fatigues you a lot, you may feel quite tired in the second half of your workouts when you hit your upper body
- You have to spend a lot of time warming up all of your separate muscles, meaning your sessions can be quite long
- Can be slightly confusing, as you may not know how to vary your full body workouts throughout the week

How To Structure Your Week

2. 3 days a week

If you would like to dedicate 3 days a week to the gym, I would also stick with full body workouts. If you do 3 of them a week, you will fall into the optimal frequency range of hitting each muscle between 2 and 4 days a week. If you decide to do this, I would recommend that you get all 3 workouts done between Monday and Friday, leaving a day's rest in between each workout. This will look like:

Monday: Full Body
Tuesday: Rest
Wednesday: Full Body
Thursday: Rest
Friday: Full Body
Saturday: Rest
Sunday: Rest

PROS
- Still very time efficient
- You hit each muscle 3 times a week, which is awesome
- You have your weekends free for social activities
- Because you don't go to the gym that often, you will never be affected by fatigue issues
- If you miss one of your workouts then you still hit each main muscle twice a week, which is still enough to progress

CONS
- Still not that much time to incorporate many isolation movements, meaning you may develop lagging muscle groups
- Because leg training fatigues you a lot, you may feel quite tired in the second half of your workouts when you hit your upper body
- Full Body sessions can take a lot of warming up, meaning your sessions can be quite long
- Can be slightly confusing, as you may not know how to vary your full body workouts throughout the week

How To Structure Your Week

3. 4 days a week

For me personally, 4 days a week in the gym is a bit of a sweet spot. It's not enough to fatigue your central nervous system that much, but it provides you with enough time in the gym to really target certain muscle groups. If this sounds good to you, then I would recommend an upper/lower split. This is one that I have used myself a lot in the past and got great results from it. It looks something like this:

Monday: Lower Body
Tuesday: Upper Body
Wednesday: Rest
Thursday: Lower Body
Friday: Upper Body
Saturday: Rest
Sunday: Rest

P
R
O
S

- You have enough time to incorporate a lot of volume for each muscle group, which is key to driving muscle growth
- You hit each muscle twice a week, which is enough
- You have time to incorporate isolation moves, meaning that you're not that likely to develop any lagging muscle groups.
- You can still have your weekends free

C
O
N
S

- If you miss one of your workouts, you will only hit one half of your body once a week meaning you won't be in the ideal frequency range for that part of you
- Upper body workouts can take a long time to do, as you have to hit so many different parts of you
- Not all parts of your body will heal as quickly as each other, meaning some parts can still be sore heading into your second session for that part of you of the week

How To Structure Your Week

4. 5 days a week

If you would like to commit 5 days a week to the gym, I would recommend this split:

Monday: Lower Body
Tuesday: Upper Body
Wednesday: Rest
Thursday: Lower Body
Friday: Push (one half of your upper body)
Saturday: Pull (the other half of your upper body)
Sunday: Rest

P R O S

- By splitting your upper body up into two different sessions on Thursdays and Fridays, you're able to really focus on certain parts of it
- Your upper body sessions on Thursdays and Fridays will not take as long as your Tuesday upper body session, as they're broken in half
- You're putting in enough time in the gym per week to incorporate a lot of volume, which is key to your body changing

C O N S

- If you miss a workout, you may only hit a certain part of your body once, which is not in the ideal frequency range
- Not all parts of your body will heal as quickly as each other, meaning some parts can still be sore heading into your second session for that part of you of the week
- You won't have your weekends free
- If you normally go out and drink on Friday evenings, there's a chance you may not be in the mood for the Saturday workout
- The more sessions you commit to, the more likely you are to miss some
- Your upper body session on Tuesday may take a long time to do

How To Structure Your Week

5. 6 days a week

If you want to go to the gym 6 days a week, I would recommend doing a push/pull/leg split twice a week. This will look something like this:

Monday: Legs
Tuesday: Push
Wednesday: Pull
Thursday: Rest
Friday: Legs
Saturday: Push
Sunday: Pull

P R O S

- By splitting your upper body up into two different sessions, you're able to incorporate a lot of volume for this area meaning you're more likely to experience hypertrophy
- Your push and pull sessions will not take as long to get through compared to if you were to do upper body workouts
- You hit all your muscles twice a week, falling into the ideal frequency range
- You have plenty of time to incorporate a lot of volume, meaning your muscles are likely to change
- Another benefit of spending a lot of time in the gym is that you are not that likely to develop any lagging muscle groups

C O N S

- If you miss a workout, you will only hit a certain part of yourself once a week, which is not in the ideal frequency range
- Not all parts of your body will heal as quickly as each other, meaning some parts can still be sore heading into your second session for that part of you of the week
- Takes up a lot of your weekend time
- If you're quite a social person, it may be hard to motivate yourself enough to go to the gym on Saturdays and Sundays
- Extremely time consuming
- Can lead to central nervous system fatigue issues, as you have to be in the gym most days of the week which can tire you out

How To Structure Your Week

FAQ's

1. How do I incorporate cardio into my week?

The great thing about cardio is that it can pretty much be incorporated anywhere in your week. As it's a different stimulus to weight training, the guidelines that you follow aren't anywhere near as strict. In contrast to weight training, you can do cardio multiple days in a row quite easily. Even though you can also do this with weights, it's much harder to do, and you need to program your sessions more carefully. So, if you're looking to build your cardiovascular fitness, you can do cardio at any time. You can even do it twice a day if you want. But make sure that you listen to your body. If your body feels drained, it might be time to take a rest day.

2. Does it matter if I hit the same body part two days in a row?

In the vast majority of cases, I would say that this is a bad idea. If you try to train your muscles two days in a row, the second day will be a lot harder than the first. Your muscles might be feeling more tired, stiff, or sore. If this is the case, it will be harder to achieve progressive overload in the gym. And if this is the case, you will not be able to force your body to change as much.

3. How long should I stick with my workout routine?

I would recommend sticking to your workout routine for 2 to 4 months at a time. If you program hop and only stick to a workout routine for a couple of weeks then progressive overload will be too hard to achieve. This is because too many variables are constantly changing when you do this. This means that it's too hard for you to know what you need to do each session to progress.

CLIENT SPOTLIGHT
IT'S NEVER TOO LATE!

JIM Lorry Driver Portsmouth, UK

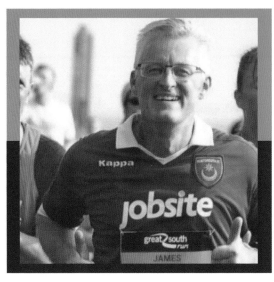

Jim initially joined a gym because he got a small health scare from his doctor. Instead of hopping on pharmaceutical medication, he wanted to take the natural route to improve his health. This involved cleaning up his diet, and joining a gym!

Despite being in his fifties, Jim had never been to a gym before. Because of this, he had no idea what to do! So he decided to come to me for help.

The priority was to put Jim on a plan that would allow him to lose weight. This would dramatically improve his health, and it did!

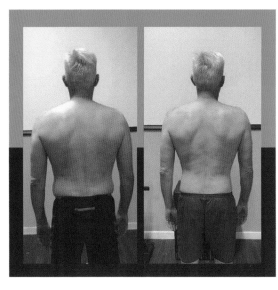

In four months, Jim lost one and a half stone. His new diet was completely different from his old one, and he got into a routine of consistently going to the gym. As a result, his health had never been better!

This shows that it's never too late to join a gym and start to work on yourself.

CHAPTER 11:
HOW TO STRUCTURE YOUR WORKOUTS

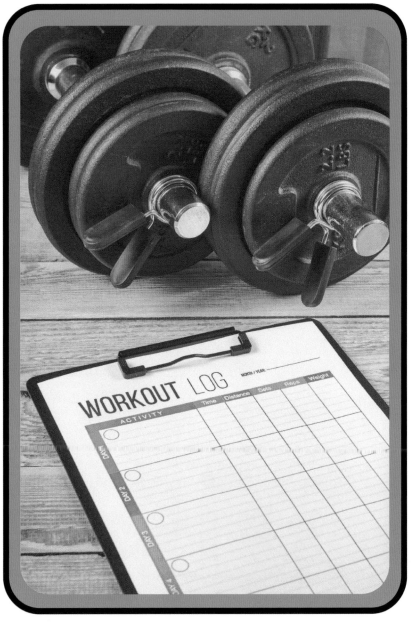

How To Structure Your Workouts

If you want to achieve great results in the gym, then structuring your workouts correctly is important. Not doing this correctly is one of the main reasons why people fail. Learning how to do this right, however, can be tricky and time-consuming.

As I've previously mentioned, many people such as myself learned what to do through a long process of trial and error. I've even spoken to people who have numerous years' worth of experience in the gym and they still don't program their sessions correctly. There are also plenty of people who don't program their sessions at all! This baffles me. As the saying goes, if you fail to plan then you plan to fail. Unfortunately, the majority of people fall into one of these two categories, meaning they never achieve great results.

Because there is not a 'one size fits all' approach when it comes to the gym, I won't be able to tell you how to make the perfect workout. Everyone will do different workouts depending on their schedules, genetics, goals, etc. However, in this section, I'll go over the most common types of workouts that you can do. With each one, I'll tell you certain points that you need to remember. I'll also give you a rough guideline that you can follow for each! Make sure you also refer back to your exercise library so you know what exercises you can include in each workout.

How To Structure Your Workouts

1) A general fitness workout

If your goal is to improve your general fitness, then you should try to incorporate a mix of cardio, weights and mobility work. This will give you a basic ability in each of the main areas of fitness, and you will still be able to change how your body looks over time too.

If you want to improve your CV fitness the most, you should do cardio first. If you want to prioritise muscle gain or weight loss more, then you should do weight training first. This is because you'll typically be worse doing the second part of the workout, as you'll be more tired. Imagine running on a treadmill after doing multiple sets of lunges and squats. The fatigue in your legs will mean that they won't be able to perform optimally. Now imagine the second scenario. Imagine you want to do your squats and lunges, but do an intense treadmill run first. If you do this, you will deplete your legs of available energy. This means that they won't feel as strong when you do your sets, making it harder to achieve progressive overload. So, if general fitness is your goal then you need to establish your priorities first. On the next page, I've given you some rough guidelines to follow if this is the type of workout that you'd like to do.

How To Structure Your Workouts

1) A general fitness workout: a rough guideline

If your CV fitness is your main goal:

Part 1 (Warm Up, 5-10 minutes): I would recommend doing a full body dynamic stretching routine and a gentle bit of cardio, such as a light uphill walk.

Part 2 (Main Body, 40-50 minutes): First off I would do 20-25 minutes of cardio. This could be HIIT training, or hopping on some CV equipment. After this, I would do 20-25 minutes of weights. This would include 4 compound exercises. Between these exercises, you should hit both your legs and your upper body.

Part 3 (Cool Down, 5-10 minutes): I would recommend doing a full body static stretching routine.

If your main goal is either strength, building muscle or losing fat:

Part 1 (Warm Up, 5-10 minutes): I would recommend doing a full body dynamic stretching routine and a gentle bit of cardio, such as a light uphill walk.

Part 2 (Main Body, 40-50 minutes): First off I would do 20-25 minutes of weights. This would include 4 compound exercises. Between these exercises, you should hit both your legs and your upper body. After this, I would do 20-25 minutes of cardio. This could be HIIT training, or hopping on some CV equipment.

Part 3 (Cool Down, 5-10 minutes): I would recommend doing a full body static stretching routine.

How To Structure Your Workouts

2) A cardiovascular workout

The good news is, you don't need a rigid structure with a CV workout like you would with a weight training one. This means that you can be flexible with what you do.

If you mainly do HIIT training, you can get through a workout in a shorter period. This means that you won't have to stay in the gym for that long. If you do low intensity cardio on a piece of equipment, this will take a lot longer to do. Both types of cardio have benefits. It's up to you which option you would like to take.

You also don't need a huge amount of variety when it comes to cardio. With weight training, it has to be extremely specific. This is because you need to program your sessions to make sure that you target every part of yourself, with adequate volume and frequency. With a CV session though, you can in theory just stay on one piece of equipment for the whole session. Alternatively, you can hop between a few different machines. If you're training for a specific event, like a marathon, then I'd say the first option is better for you. If you're someone who does like variety though, then I would recommend bouncing between a few different pieces of cardio equipment in a session. This is just to prevent you from becoming too bored.

How To Structure Your Workouts

2) A cardiovascular workout: a rough guideline

Part 1 (Warm Up, 5-10 minutes): I would recommend doing a full body dynamic stretching routine. You can also do a gentle bit of cardio, such as a light uphill walk, if you want to. However, make sure the intensity of your warm up is very different to the intensity of what you do afterwards.

Part 2 (Main Body, 40-50 minutes): As discussed, there are several different ways you can program this session. A really simple way though is just 10 minutes on the treadmill followed by 10 minutes on the bicycle, rower and cross trainer.

Part 3 (Cool Down, 5-10 minutes): I would recommend doing a full body static stretching routine.

How To Structure Your Workouts

3) A weights workout: full body with a rough guideline

As previously discussed, full body workouts are awesome. They just have so many benefits. The key point to remember here is to obviously make sure that you work most of your main muscles. It doesn't have to be an even split though. For instance, you can do a full body workout that consists of legs for the first 25% of it, and then upper body for the remaining 75%. It's up to you.

Try to mainly prioritise the compound lifts though, as these are the best at changing your body. Afterwards, finish off with some isolation exercises. Make sure that you also hit your legs first, then finish off with upper body. Here's what that might look like:

Part 1 (Warm Up, 5-10 minutes): I would recommend doing a full body dynamic stretching routine. You can also do a gentle bit of cardio, such as a light uphill walk.

Part 2 (Main Body, 40-50 minutes): A rough workout structure that you can follow starts with you doing 3 leg exercises. Make sure at least 2 of them are compound lifts. Afterwards, do 3 upper body exercises. Make at least 2 of them compound lifts too. You can also do 1 core exercise to finish off.

Part 3 (Cool Down, 5-10 minutes): I would recommend doing a full body static stretching routine.

How To Structure Your Workouts

4) A weights workout: legs with a rough guideline

If you looked at 100 different peoples' leg sessions then they would all probably look completely different, and I can see why. In truth, there are plenty of different leg exercises that you can do, and in different orders.

When you program your leg sessions, you just need to make sure that you hit your quadriceps, hamstrings and glutes. Too many people focus just on their quadriceps. This will leave a lot of imbalances between the front side of their body and the back side of their body. Also, make sure that you incorporate at least one single-legged exercise for balance and stability. Here's a rough guideline for you to follow:

Part 1 (Warm Up, 5-10 minutes): I would recommend doing a full body dynamic stretching routine. You can also do a gentle bit of cardio. If you do this, I would recommend the bicycle.

Part 2 (Main Body, 40-50 minutes): In this workout, try to incorporate at least 3 or 4 compound exercises. After doing these, leg extensions and leg curls are great to do afterwards to burn your thighs more. You also have the option of finishing with a core exercise.

Part 3 (Cool Down, 5-10 minutes): I would recommend doing a full body static stretching routine.

How To Structure Your Workouts

5) A weights workout: upper body with a rough guideline

There isn't a strict way to program your upper body sessions, as there are plenty of exercises that you can choose. However, programming your upper body sessions can be harder than programming your leg sessions. This is because there are far more muscles to hit in your upper body sessions, and you need to make sure that you hit most of them. The main muscles that you need to hit are your chest, back, shoulders, triceps and biceps. It would also typically go in that order, as you want to work the bigger muscles first. Here's a rough guideline for you to follow:

Part 1 (Warm Up, 5-10 minutes): I would recommend doing an upper body dynamic stretching routine. You can also do a gentle bit of cardio. If you do this, I would recommend the rower.

Part 2 (Main Body, 40-50 minutes): In this workout, try to start with at least 3 or 4 compound exercises. After doing these, try to incorporate some isolation moves for your shoulders and arms. Some good choices would be side raises, rear delt flies, bicep curls or tricep extensions. There's also the potential to finish off with a core exercise.

Part 3 (Cool Down, 5-10 minutes): I would recommend doing a full body static stretching routine.

How To Structure Your Workouts

6) A weights workout: a pull workout with a rough guideline

Pull workouts can be great at providing you with sufficient volume to grow half of your main upper body muscles. With this type of workout, you need to try to incorporate exercises that work your traps, midback, lats, shoulders and biceps. You can find these exercises in the back, shoulder, and arm sections of your exercise library. Here's a rough guideline that you can follow:

Part 1 (Warm Up, 5-10 minutes): I would recommend doing an upper body dynamic stretching routine. You can also do a gentle bit of cardio. If you do this, I would recommend the rower.

Part 2 (Main Body, 40-50 minutes): In this workout, try to start with at least 3 or 4 compound exercises. After doing these, try to incorporate some isolation moves for your shoulders and arms. Some good choices would be rear delt flies and bicep curls. There's also the potential to finish off with a core exercise.

Part 3 (Cool Down, 5-10 minutes): I would recommend doing a full body static stretching routine.

How To Structure Your Workouts

7) A weights workout: a push workout with a rough guideline

Push workouts can be great at providing you with sufficient volume to grow half of your main upper body muscles. With this type of workout, you need to incorporate exercises that work your chest, shoulders and triceps. You can find these exercises in the chest, shoulder, and arm sections of your exercise library. Here's what that would look like:

Part 1 (Warm Up, 5-10 minutes): I would recommend doing an upper body dynamic stretching routine. You can also do a gentle bit of cardio. If you do this, I would recommend the rower.

Part 2 (Main Body, 40-50 minutes): In this workout, try to start with at least 3 or 4 compound exercises. After doing these, try to incorporate some isolation moves for your shoulders and arms. Some good choices would be side raises and tricep extensions. There's also the potential to finish off with a core exercise.

Part 3 (Cool Down, 5-10 minutes): I would recommend doing a full body static stretching routine.

How To Structure Your Workouts

FAQ's

1. Does the exercise order matter?

In most cases, whatever exercise you do negatively impacts the next exercise after that. Because of that, you normally want to get the harder and heavier movements out of the way first. If you do this, your muscles and central nervous system will be in a fresher state to perform those exercises. And if that's the case, then you're more likely to work hard and progress in those lifts. Imagine doing the hardest exercise last! You may not even have the energy to perform it correctly, let alone progress with it!

2. You haven't mentioned core work much, where do I incorporate it?

Many people believe that you should train your core differently than all your other muscles. This doesn't make any sense though. The muscles in your core are very similar to other muscles in your body, thus meaning they should be trained in the same way. This means that you should hit them between 2 and 4 times a week, and you should also do between 10 and 20 total sets for your core per week. Like with your other muscles, I would recommend giving yourself at least a day's rest before hitting your core again.

In terms of how to structure your core training, there are plenty of different ways to go about it. You could do 4 sets at the end of each of your 3 full-body workouts a week, meaning you fall into that 10-20 total weekly sets range. Alternatively, you could just pick 2 of your weekly workouts and do 5-10 sets at the end of both workouts. The choice is yours. However, I would normally do core work last in a workout. This is because it doesn't take that much energy to do.

How To Structure Your Workouts

3.   What happens if the machine that I want to use is taken?

This is a problem that you'll encounter quite frequently, especially if you're in the gym at busier times. In this situation, you have two options. The first is that you can try to find a similar exercise to what you're meant to be doing and do that instead. For example, let's say that you are meant to be doing a barbell back squat, but all of the squat racks are taken. Instead, you can do a kettlebell goblet squat. The next time you do this session though, make sure that you go back to the originally planned exercise.

The second option is that you just move onto the next exercise. When you've done that, you go back to what you were supposed to be doing. Both options are fine.

4.   Should compound moves always come first?

Typically speaking, compound exercises should come first. This is because compound exercises are typically better at changing your body compared to isolation movements. Therefore, you want to go into these types of sets in a fresher state.

This isn't always the case though. In some cases, doing isolation movements before a compound move can be helpful. For instance, doing leg curls before deadlifts can get more blood in your hamstrings. Then when you do the deadlifts, your hamstrings are more likely to be engaged in that lift.

CHAPTER 12:
OVERCOMING YOUR ISSUES

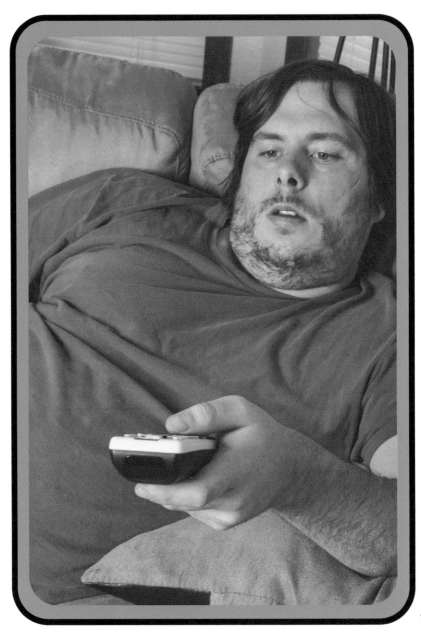

Overcoming Your Issues

Now, it's all very well knowing what to do in the gym, but this still doesn't guarantee that you'll actually be consistent. This is because we're not robots! We're human. And as humans, our decisions are largely influenced by both our internal and external problems. For this reason, unless you're a dedicated professional athlete, it's extremely unlikely that you'll be consistent 100% of the time. So don't beat yourself up if you miss some workouts! Just accept that this will happen and aim to get straight back on the wagon as soon as possible.

Having said that, there are still certain things that you can do to try to maintain your consistency in tougher times. In this section, I'll take you through the most common problems that you may experience in your fitness journey. Better yet, in each one, I'll even tell you the best ways to combat them. Let's go!

1. A lack of motivation

Earlier on in this book, I told you that it's completely normal to have motivation dips. Yes, it would be a lot easier to be consistent if you were able to stay motivated all the time. In reality though, this will never be the case. For me, I reckon I'm only motivated for around 25% of my workouts. This is again because motivation is just a temporary feeling that comes and goes. So, if you are looking for motivation, please stop, as this is a waste of time. Follow these 7 tips instead!

Overcoming Your Issues

1) Focus on enjoying the journey

If you're at a point in your journey where you're not progressing as you'd like to, it's easy to become frustrated. And when you feel frustrated, you may look for shortcuts. For example, let's say you want to lose 2 stone, and maybe you haven't lost any weight for a month. What some people might do at this point is implement over the top methods to speed up their progress, such as a juice fast or not eating altogether. There are many reasons why this is a terrible idea, one of which is the fact that these methods aren't sustainable. And if that's the case, you're not going to be able to maintain that lifestyle for very long before becoming miserable.

So, one of the best pieces of advice I can give you is this: try to focus on building a lifestyle that you can sustain and enjoy rather than focusing on rushing to the end result. Make sure you do what you must do regularly, but make sure that it's not so over the top to the point that you can't carry it on for very long. There's no need to kill yourself in the gym 7 days a week when you can make great progress only going 3-4 days a week.

So please try to focus on enjoying the process. If you do that, it's more likely that you'll be able to stay consistent with everything that you need to do in the long run. Remember, the person who loves walking will always walk further than the person who loves the destination! So please, have some patience.

Overcoming Your Issues

2) Change your indicator of success

This is another useful tool that you can use if you find your motivation levels starting to dip. Let's say that you're trying to build some muscle, but your motivation levels are dipping as you aren't seeing any physical changes in yourself yet. Instead of just looking at yourself in the mirror more, shift your mindset and focus on another indicator of success instead. In this case, it would be useful to focus on if you're hitting more personal bests in the gym. As previously mentioned, PB's lead to progressive overload. And progressive overload leads to physical changes in your body. So, if you're not seeing any muscle gains yet, but you are hitting PB's, this a sign that you are actually moving in the right direction. The great thing about the gym is it's very easy to quantify things. If you go from bicep curling 5kg for 8 reps, to 10 reps, and the form is as good, then you're 100% moving in the right direction. You cannot in any way deny this.

Therefore, it's important to shift your indicator of success sometimes. If you don't, then you're not looking at the bigger picture and could think that you're not moving in the right direction when you actually are.

3) Celebrate your wins

Regardless of your rate of progress, your motivation levels will go up and down anyway. This is because motivation is a temporary feeling, just like feeling tired when you wake up. Temporary feelings like this will always come and go. Therefore, don't panic if you find yourself lacking motivation at times!

However, if you're in need of short term bursts of motivation to pick yourself up again, then celebrating your wins is a great thing to do. This can be done in a lot of different ways, with the most common one being reminding yourself of all the PB's that you've hit this week! When you do this, you will feel proud of yourself. This will in turn lead to you becoming more motivated.

Overcoming Your Issues

4) Visual imagination

Visual imagination is a powerful tool that we can use to shape our lives. If you want your body to physically change, you can imagine yourself down the line with the body that you desire. The main thing to think about here isn't the result itself, but rather how the result makes you feel. For instance, let's say that you want to lose weight, but your motivation levels are starting to dip. In this case, try to envision your future slimmer self and all those positive feelings that come with your new look. For example, this could be your new found confidence. When we envision those feelings, it means that we're more likely to experience them for real in the future.

5) Habit stacking

Habit stacking is an unbelievably effective tactic to increase your levels of consistency, regardless of how you feel at a particular time. Habit stacking involves pairing a task that you want to do, with a task that you already do every day. For instance, let's say that you want to plan to go to the gym in the mornings. After that, you need to think about tasks that you do in the morning every single day without fail. Brushing your teeth could be a good choice. After you've done this, you need to make sure that you leave for the gym after you brush your teeth every day. So after you brush your teeth, you get changed into your gym gear and you step out of the door. Sooner or later, this association will become second nature. So, every time you do brush your teeth, your brain will automatically think that it's time to go to the gym. When the process becomes this automatic, it won't matter if you're feeling unmotivated or not. The outcome will still be the same: you will go to the gym.

Overcoming Your Issues

6) Adding accountability

Out of every point that I've mentioned so far, this is by far the most effective solution. I won't go into too much detail now, as I'm going to talk about this in more detail towards the end of this book. But having a PT or a coach in your corner makes such a difference. You're less likely to struggle with consistency with someone in your corner as you will not want to let them down, as well as yourself.

Overcoming Your Issues

2. The fear of getting too bulky

Within my 5 years in this industry, I've spoken to hundreds of women who have had this fear. So many women believe that they shouldn't lift weights because they'll get huge muscles if they do. This is a big problem. Because weight training is actually the best form of training for weight loss. So not only is this fear completely irrational, but it's also very detrimental too. If you're currently in this boat, here are my top tips to combat this issue.

1) Acknowledge the facts

If you properly learn what you have to do to build muscle, this should ease your fears of lifting weights. You don't get big by accident. In fact, so many people work hard to build muscle and still can't build very much at all. This is because building muscle is a slow, hard process. It takes years and years of doing the right things consistently to get that type of body. It won't happen by simply lifting some weights for a couple of months. I would like you to keep in mind what I said earlier on in this book to validate my point. In terms of weight loss, you can typically look to lose 0.5lbs-1.5lbs a week. But you'd be extremely lucky in most cases to build that amount of muscle in a month. The speed of progress is just not the same.

Overcoming Your Issues

You should also understand that to get big, you have to eat big. Think of building muscle kind of like building a house. Yes, it's possible to build a big house just like how you can build big muscles. But to do that, you need loads of materials. A house can never get built if there aren't enough bricks to build it! And it's the same thing with your muscles. If you don't consume enough calories, then you physically don't have the raw materials available to build muscles of that size.

Of course, there are some exceptions. If you're someone who is new to lifting weights, you can still build muscle when you don't eat that many calories. The only other exception is when you have extremely good genetics. This can warrant you progressing very quickly even if you don't do things completely right. However, it's more than likely that you won't fall into this category, as most of us don't!

2) Ease yourself in

If you've read the paragraph above and you still have a bit of a mental barrier, I would recommend going to some gym classes for the time being. It is extremely unlikely that you will get muscles from going to gym classes. Even the ones that involve you lifting weights don't provide you with a strong muscle building stimulus. That might sound unusual to some of you. But the reality is, these types of classes are still cardio based. In gym classes, you have to do almost endless reps for 30-45 minutes. The only way to do this is by lifting extremely light weights, so you are capable of lifting them for such a long period of time. Because the weight is so light and some of the other muscle building parameters are missing as well, you won't grow big muscles.

Alternatively, proper weight training which does lead to muscle growth involves much heavier, much more intense exercise. To initiate a muscle building response, you have to work hard in a set to the point where you physically need to rest for at least a minute before continuing. In a class, this doesn't happen.

Overcoming Your Issues

This is, again, because the training involves much lighter weight, which means you can keep doing it for much longer periods of time.

So, if you are still a bit worried about lifting weights, I would say that initially going to classes is a good idea for you. They're less intense but also provide you with some experience in lifting weights. This will make it easier for you to transition to the gym floor afterwards.

<u>3. Gym Anxiety</u>

Gym anxiety is a very real thing. Out of everybody that I speak to, this is maybe the most common issue that comes up. But just because your gym anxiety is real, doesn't mean that it can't be fixed (or at least limited.) In fact, I know so many good methods that will really help to alleviate these feelings for you. So don't worry, I've got you! Let's dive in!

1) Get to know the staff members

This is something that you can do that will get you feeling a lot more comfortable in the gym. If you know, like, and trust the people who work at the gym then naturally you feel a lot less anxious there. So, I know it can be tough, but try your best to talk to the staff when you can.

Overcoming Your Issues

2) Hire a PT

Leading on from that last point, having a trainer by your side is probably the most effective way to alleviate your gym anxiety. If you do have someone by your side, you won't worry that people are watching you do anything wrong. If you build a good relationship with your PT on top, then you will look forward to your gym sessions more and become a lot more comfortable in the gym.

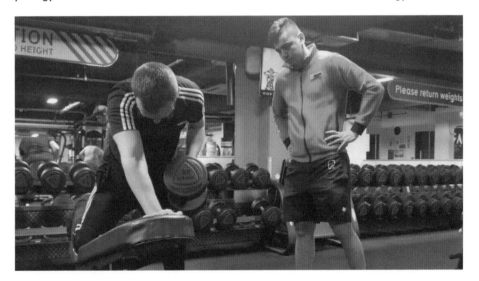

3) Work out in a quieter area

While the free weights area is a great place for you to progress, it's the area of the gym that's most likely to make you anxious. This is partly because you'll often find more experienced and knowledgeable people in this area. When this is the case, you might be more worried about being watched. The free weights area also involves you doing more technical lifts. If you don't have faith in yourself to perform them correctly, then you will naturally feel more anxious trying to perform them. Due to these reasons, I think that it's best to somewhat limit your time in this area if you are a beginner with some anxiety issues.

Overcoming Your Issues

4) Go during quieter times

This is a great tactic to ease your nerves. If there are more people in the gym, you'll natural feel more anxious. So as long as your lifestyle allows it, try to go during quieter times. Quieter times in gyms are typically during mid-morning, and mid-afternoon on a weekday. If you are going to have weekend sessions, try going early morning or late evening.

5) Find a gym buddy

There are plenty of reasons why having a gym buddy can be beneficial! If you get on with your gym buddy, you will feel a lot more comfortable in the gym with them by your side.

One thing I would say, is make sure that your gym partner is reliable. If you have gym anxiety and you rely on someone who is flaky, it's likely that you'll consider skipping your session if they bail. So, choose wisely! If you don't, you might become even less consistent than you would otherwise.

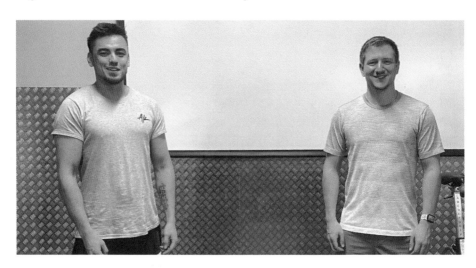

Overcoming Your Issues

4. A Lack of confidence

A lack of confidence is easily linked with gym anxiety. Therefore, all the methods in the section above will also be helpful to correct this problem too.

Also, try to acknowledge the fact that this can easily change with time once you gain more knowledge about what you're doing. If you follow the advice that I've given you in this book, your confidence can change a hell of a lot! As I've mentioned to you already, this is what I've personally experienced myself. It can happen! You just have to try to do the right things as consistently as possible. If you do this, your faith and belief in yourself will change over time.

5. Injuries

If you have injuries that are stopping you from going to the gym, you should go to see a proper professional who specialises in rehabilitation. Rehab can be very confusing, especially if you don't have much experience at the gym. Therefore, injuries are not something you should try to fix yourself. So, save yourself a bunch of time and get some specific exercises that will aid you in your recovery.

Although PT's will have some basic knowledge in this area, I wouldn't recommend going to see one about an injury. This is because they specialise in training and body transformations, not rehab. Some might try to blag it, so you pay them some money. I know it's convenient to take them up on this but try to refrain. It's better to see someone who's an expert in that specific field.

Overcoming Your Issues

6. Don't enjoy the gym

1) Incorporate the type of exercise that you enjoy the most

There's no denying that some types of exercise are just better for you if you want to achieve certain things. Having said that, it wouldn't hurt to just start with the activities that you prefer. That way, you're less likely to bail on your gym sessions.

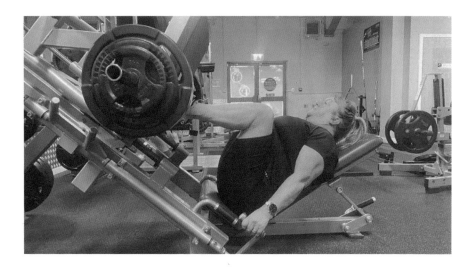

2) Focus on increasing your numbers

Typically, we enjoy things that we're good at. On the other side of the spectrum, we dislike things that we're not good at. For instance, I can't stand cricket. But that's mainly because I'm not good at catching balls! So logically speaking, we should look to improve at something if we want to enjoy it more.

Overcoming Your Issues

To make sure this is the case, you need to focus on progressive overload and increasing your numbers as often as you can. Once this happens then you'll start to believe in yourself more and also become prouder of yourself for what you're achieving. As your ability in this department goes up, I guarantee that you will start to enjoy the gym a hell of a lot more!

7. Worrying that people are watching you

This one is a common fear amongst people with minimal gym experience. It's all very well for me to tell you that this doesn't happen as much as you think. In reality though, me saying this won't do much to ease your mind. So instead, here are my top strategies to work around this issue:

1) Work out in a quieter area

If you work out in an area of the gym where there are fewer people, naturally this will bring you more peace of mind. Two good places to work out are either in the stretching area or in the studio if there isn't a class on at the time!

2) Be in your own world

If you worry that people are watching you in the gym, try to go to the gym with two items. The first one is a set of headphones. When you listen to music that you enjoy, this will not only ease your worries but also lets you divert your attention to other things. The second thing that I would recommend is wearing a hoodie, with your hood up. If you have a hood covering your face, this will make you feel safer in this environment.

Overcoming Your Issues

8. Feeling disappointed about your lack of progress

Maybe you won't progress as quickly as you'd like to. Or maybe you will, but you'll struggle to identify the progress that you've made. Either way, in most cases, we are our own biggest critics. If you feel disappointed at any point in your journey, here are two great ways to reduce these negative feelings:

1) Practice acceptance

You don't necessarily experience a lack of happiness because of the point that you're at. But rather, you experience a lack of happiness from not fully accepting the point you're at. So, practicing acceptance is one of the most effective methods to lead to you being content about your body and your life in general. Therefore, it is so important that you accept the fact that progress may take you longer than you might like. Doing so will minimize the rush that you'll feel to achieve that progress. In turn, this will reduce the pressure that you put yourself under. But as long as you keep doing everything that you can to move forward, you will get there in the end anyway!

2) Celebrate your wins

This can not only help you deal with a lack of motivation, but also help you deal with a lack of disappointment in yourself too. When you take a step back and acknowledge what you have accomplished, rather than what you have not, then you'll feel more proud of yourself. A lot of the time our negative emotions can blind us from the progress that we are actually making. Don't let that happen to you!

CLIENT SPOTLIGHT
GUIDANCE IS EVERYTHING!

KYLE Scientist Boston, USA

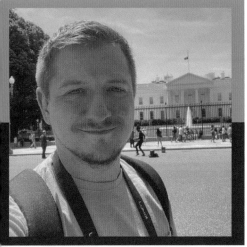

Kyle has had every body you can think of. At first, he was unhealthily thin. Next, he became overweight. Lastly, he developed a bit of a 'dad bod.' The thing is, though, he did work out earlier in his life, he just didn't exactly know what he should be doing!

After we connected on Instagram, Kyle asked for my help, saying it was time that he got some professional guidance.

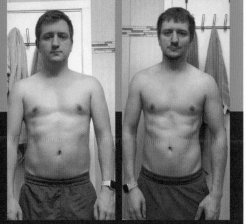

The result is that he genuinely got into the best shape of his life within just three months. He finally had that six-pack that he always wanted, and his confidence grew so much because of this. To this day, Kyle is still putting in the work and getting into better shape every month.

I always hear people say that they can "do it alone." The reality is, however, that you will always do better with someone in your corner due to the guidance and accountability that they can provide.

If you've been trying to get in shape on your own for a while now with no results, this could be a great option for you.

CHAPTER 13:
THE GAME CHANGER

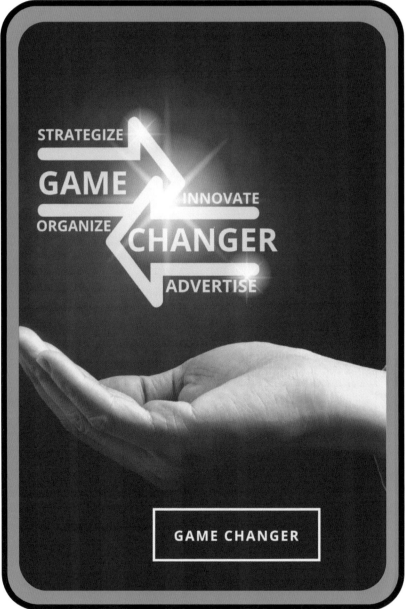

THE GAME CHANGER

I hope by now that you feel 10x more confident about going to the gym than you did before you started reading this book. There's no doubt that the knowledge that you will have gained will help you in leaps and bounds. Now, it's important to talk about something that will really make the difference: getting extra support.

Many people have the impression that the only benefit that you gain from having a coach in your corner is the knowledge that you can gain from them. Because of this, many people who feel like they have a good degree of knowledge think that they don't need a coach. Gaining knowledge is only one aspect of coaching though and thinking like this means that you have a very minimalistic view. If you really tried hard enough, and long enough, you could research the correct information that you need on google. While getting a coach can give you the information that you need at a quicker rate than that, there are so many more layers to coaching than just gaining knowledge.

I always say that knowing what to do is one thing, but actually doing it is something completely different. You already know that you should be going to the gym more. You already know that you would benefit from reducing your alcohol consumption. You already know that you would benefit from eating healthier. But the question is, are you actually doing these things? Earlier in this book I gave you a bunch of ideas on how to be more consistent when going to the gym. I hope that these ideas help you. But the reality is that just because you now know something, doesn't mean that you'll implement that piece of knowledge.

And that's exactly where coaching comes in. While there are many layers of coaching, the main benefit of having someone there is the accountability that you gain. With someone in your corner, you're far more likely to follow through with what you say you're going to do. This is partly because you want to stick to your word, and partly because you don't want to disappoint your coach with false promises. Unfortunately, using a friend or a family member doesn't quite have the same effect. To experience truly effective levels of accountability you need to involve a third party, someone completely unrelated to you.

THE GAME CHANGER

While I do have a lot of knowledge that my online clients benefit from, I don't feel like that's the main reason why they do well. The reason that they do so well is because of the high levels of accountability that I provide. All online coaches do things differently, so it's hard for me to outline the exact features typically involved when working with someone. With me though, I normally check in with my online clients via whatsapp. We also have one weekly zoom catch up call where we talk about how their week has gone. I also get them to connect their Fitbit and MyFitnessPal app to a website so I can see what their activity and diet is like, at any time. Because of these things, my clients know that they must stay on track. They know that I'm always watching what they do, and they know that they must be consistent because I check in with them so frequently. This degree of accountability means that they're far more likely to follow through with what they say they're going to do, and therefore be more consistent because of that.

This is why plenty of coaches like myself have also gotten help in the past. It's not necessarily that we need to gain a lot more knowledge about things. It's that we need someone in our corner to hold us accountable too. A few years ago, I reached out to someone for help. When I spoke to some of my clients and friends about this, some of them were shocked. Some of them assumed that I asked for help because I lacked knowledge. This is a very bad mindset to have though. It wasn't that I didn't know enough, but it was because I wasn't consistent enough with doing what I needed to do to hit my goals. I knew that adding in a layer of accountability would help, and it did. If I didn't do what I was meant to do, that person asked why. After I felt that disappointment if I let him down, I would get my act together. Therefore in that period, I honestly progressed quicker than any other time of my life.

Because of my own experience, and my clients' experiences, I know how much of a difference the power of accountability can make. It's honestly a game changer. So if you do struggle with consistency, this is by far the best route that you can go down. You will also learn a lot along the way.

CHAPTER 14:
FINAL THOUGHTS

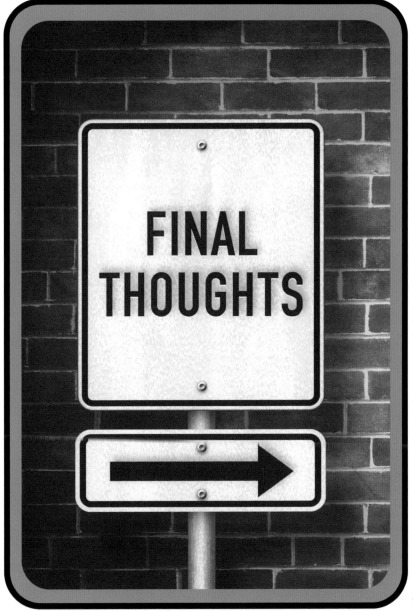

FINAL THOUGHTS

This book took me a long time to write, so I really appreciate that you've put in the time to read it all. Doing this will put you lightyears ahead of other beginners who haven't actively gone out of their way to get some help. So well done!

One of the last things that I want to say to you is that despite gaining all this knowledge, the first few weeks in the gym will still be hard for you. If you haven't built a routine of consistently going, it may be hard for you to find the willpower to initially go. This is especially the case because you're yet to experience any real progress, and making progress motivates you to keep going. So, I'm not going to lie, you may have to really drag yourself to the gym for the first few weeks.

However, this won't be forever. It may be hard for you to envision now, but you will genuinely get to a point where it's harder for you to not go than it is to go. This is because once you see the progress that you can make and the benefits that you can experience, it's hard to stop. If you play your cards right, you will truly become addicted to the process of self-improvement. So, hang in there and don't give up.

FINAL THOUGHTS

Lastly, I want you to know that I'm here to help. If you think you could benefit from having me in your corner, feel free to contact me using one of the methods below. I would be happy to have a chat with you about my coaching and how it can help you. I know the process of getting in shape can be long, confusing and overwhelming. I want to make sure that the journey is as smooth as possible for you, and coaching is the best way to stop these things from happening! But even if you don't fancy getting paid help, I'm still here for you. If you need any advice, don't hesitate to get in touch with me. I've got you!

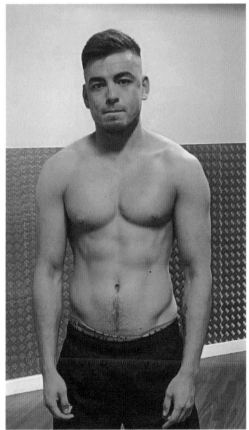

WhatsApp: +447787166065
Email: aaronchoi@weightlossworldwideltd.com
Instagram: @aaronchoi_pt
Facebook: https://www.facebook.com/weightlossworldwideltd

Printed in Great Britain
by Amazon

37081924R00096